The
Able Life
of
Cody Jane

The
Able Life
of
Cody Jane

Still Celebrating

MARLY CORNELL

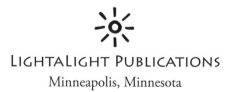

LightaLight Publications
Minneapolis, Minnesota

LightaLight Publications
Minneapolis, Minnesota

LightaLightPublications.com

Cover design by Bookwrights
Cover photos by Dennis Ahlburg
Interior by Dorie McClelland

Some names have been changed to protect privacy.

Scripture quotations from *The Living Bible.* Wheaton: Tyndale House, 1980,
c1971 by Tyndale House Publishers, Inc. Used by permission.
All rights reserved.

ISBN 978-0-9831777-0-8
Library of Congress Control Number: 2010919218

Printed in the United States of America

To all those living on the ragged edge

Contents

For he orders his angels to protect you wherever you go.
They will steady you with their hands to keep you
from stumbling against the rocks on the trail.

Psalm 91:11–12
The Living Bible

Foreword

When I began training in neurosurgery the aggressive treatment of babies born with myelomeningocele was still a relatively new idea. Prominent pediatricians and neurosurgeons still had serious discussions about the ethics of treating these children, and experience with adults with myelomeningocele and hydrocephalus was limited. If they had known Cody Jane Ahlburg, the discussion would have been very different.

Cody filled any room she was in. There was no doubt who was in charge. She was smart enough to take control of her life, insist on the care that she needed, and wise enough to accept the advice of those who could provide the specialized care she required. She was, indeed, unforgettable.

Her story is not just one of courage, humor, and refusal to be defeated by serious medical disorders, but also of the multiple medical problems that ultimately ended her life. The condition we call spina bifida affects more than just the spine. The nervous system of a person with myelomeningocele has many abnormalities that can cause difficulty at different times in life. With aggressive treatment our patients have grown up with us, and our experience with the many different manifestations of nervous system dysfunction that adults with spina bifida may encounter is rapidly increasing. The accumulation of problems over time carries significant risks and may ultimately shorten life.

Each of us has limitations that we wish we did not have. If we could face them with the same degree of acceptance, combined with refusal to let them impose unnecessary limitations, that Cody demonstrated, we would live richer and fuller lives, no matter how long we lived them.

Stephen Haines, MD
Minneapolis, Minnesota

Stephen J. Haines, MD is the Lyle A. French Chair and the professor and head of the Department of Neurosurgery at the University of Minnesota.

Foreword

Who among us has not faced a barrier that seemed insurmountable? In a culture where we are all too often labeled by what we can*not* accomplish rather than by what we can do, *The Able Life of Cody Jane* serves as a reminder that life is simply too short to be defined by others' misperceptions of our abilities.

During a decade of service to the spina bifida community, I've had the pleasure of meeting thousands of seemingly ordinary people who, under the extreme pressures of this complex and challenging birth defect, lead inspiring lives. In this book we are privileged to peek through a window opened by Cody's mother, Marly Cornell, who tells the story of one such young person who lived with joy, laughter, and dignity. Cody had a zest for life and a tenacity that demonstrates all that can be achieved when one just keeps moving forward. Her encouragement of others to look beyond their preconceptions about her abilities is an inspiration to each of us.

Spina bifida can affect any family, and its complications can influence any number of systems of the body. Children born with spina bifida may face multiple surgeries before they even reach the age of eighteen, and must navigate an array of social and physical barriers in their pursuit of mobility and inclusion. Adults with spina bifida deal with a range of obstacles to a fully independent life. Obtaining adequate and accessible medical care, living accommodations, transportation, education, job training, and employment are all hard-won achievements, particularly in light of the subtle and overt forms of discrimination that are part of the life experience for anyone with a disability.

Those who continue to embrace the joy and fun in life, while struggling for those things that so many others take for granted, are passionate people whose determination and drive is humbling. Cody Jane is a shining representative of that spirit. Her amazing heart, and her resolve that she could—and would—accomplish anything she set her mind to, poignantly demonstrates the strength that lives within so many of our families. *The Able Life of Cody Jane* compels us all to live with greater courage, to embrace a life rich with humor, happiness, and love. Cody's life was truly an "able" one.

Cindy Brownstein, President and CEO
Spina Bifida Association
Washington, DC
www.spinabifidaassociation.org

Introduction

My daughter Cody was always looking for books that told her story—books that said something useful about how others aspiring for independence dealt with real-life challenges that were sometimes difficult, and oftentimes funny. We once talked about writing a book about her life. Cody wasn't convinced anyone would be interested in "some woman who's been through a lot of surgeries and junk." She did not appreciate the suggestion that she was in any way special.

Cody had no tolerance for anyone's feeling sorry for her. She wanted others to understand "how interesting living a life having to use a wheelchair can be—how the struggles of life may look horrible to the 'normal' person, but to us, we are just living—like them." Disability did not define Cody or stop her from doing what she wanted to do. She focused on love, laughter, family, fun, and helping others.

Three days before her birthday in 2003, Cody sent me this email:

> Thanks for giving birth to me, and keeping me, even though I cost so much over the last almost 32 years. A lot of parents give up on their handicapped kids. The ones that don't give up should get praised. Thank you for keeping me. Love you, too. Cody

Her thanks for "keeping" her reminded me of my mother's suggestion right after Cody was born. I recoiled at Mom's idea to place my baby in a "home." That same day, Tad's mother told him about her prayer that our child be mentally retarded rather than be aware of her birth defect and physical disability. At the time, I was horrified by these reactions. Many years passed before I realized that Cody's grandmothers both responded to her birth with protective intentions. My mother hoped to shield me from the difficulties and hardships she imagined we'd face. Tad's mother sought to protect Cody from the suffering she might endure knowing she was "defective." Thirty-two years later I still felt so much gratitude for the life of my daughter. Of course she and I were each wounded by her fear and suffering, and so was anyone else who loved her. But *far* greater than any associated pain was the absolute joy that was Cody.

I answered her email:

> You are worth every penny and every ounce of energy I have. You are the most important thing to ever happen to me, and I am the luckiest parent in the entire world. I love your guts, and I am happy that you were born almost 32 years ago. You are a gift to me that God must have loved me very much to let me have.

Chapter 1

The Importance of Dogs and Neurosurgeons

My mother suspected correctly that my main reason for marrying in the middle of my freshman year of college in 1968 was to attend the Miami Pop Festival. I wasn't allowed to take a long-distance trip with a boy. Tad suggested marriage, and I agreed. At eighteen, I was completely in love with Tad. Firmly entrenched in the sixties' counterculture, we shared ideals and considered ourselves seekers of spiritual truth and social justice. As the war in Vietnam divided the country, we embraced the peace movement and supported civil rights.

Three days after Christmas, we exchanged wedding vows in my parents' living room. Tad looked handsome in his yellow-tinted wire-rimmed glasses and "good" jacket and tie. His hair hung to his shoulders. I wore a purple minidress. Friends played guitars and a dulcimer. Our wedding gifts ranged from a toaster and a blender to homemade bread and a half-ounce bag of marijuana.

Neither of us questioned that we'd start having kids soon after college. I wanted to be a young mother. My mother was in her forties when I was born. She endured menopause and my tumultuous teen years at the same time.

Sedation during childbirth was customary in standard hospitals in Philadelphia in 1972, so Tad and I chose a maternity center where "natural" childbirth was allowed. When Cody was a small child, she never tired of hearing the story of her first few moments and the way we met. My first look at her was in an envelope of "uh oh."

Cody emerged quietly on a Sunday morning in late August after six hours of labor. The doctor cautioned not to touch the baby's lower back as the midwife carefully placed the five-pound, eight-and-one-half-ounce newborn on my stomach. The physician told me at once that my baby had a congenital birth defect called spina bifida. I asked what that meant. He said he'd get more information right away, but for now he knew she might be paralyzed or brain damaged. He paused before adding, "She might not live." He again instructed me not to touch a dime-sized pink membrane visible on the middle of her lower back.

I looked at the pale-skinned baby lying on my stomach. She was wide awake and calm. Her dark-blue eyes peered up toward my face. I reached for her hand and she grabbed my thumb. I was startled by the strength of her grip. Despite what the doctor had just said, I could see my kid was okay. From that moment Tad and I knew that whatever physical problems she might have, she was fine. She was alert. She was okay. I smiled at Cody Jane.

After a nurse took Cody away to have a protective covering placed over the small exposed area on her back, I was moved to a patient room. Tad and I waited there for a pediatrician to come and tell us more about Cody's situation. Tad called his parents and wept when his mother cried on the phone.

When the pediatrician arrived, his face was so sad I almost cried. He said Cody's legs were paralyzed. She'd been such a feisty kicker throughout my pregnancy—her arms alone must have caused all the movement I'd felt. The doctor said in a sympathetic voice, "We don't know what all might be wrong with your daughter; she might not live." He said Cody needed surgery to close the spot at the base of her spine to prevent infection, meningitis, and further nerve damage. Tad could ride the short distance downtown with her in an ambulance within the hour. Specialists at a university hospital would perform the operation that afternoon.

Cody was brought to me for a moment before they left. I held my hand next to her arm to measure it against part of me. I wanted to remember how tiny she was the day she was born. Her eyes were bright and attentive, her skin soft. I stroked her wispy golden hair and perfect ears.

After Cody and Tad left, a nurse explained that I was put in a room away from other mothers and infants "for my own good" since I was without *my* baby. That nurse was dead wrong; I felt left out.

I couldn't make a long-distance call to my parents from my room. My father had changed jobs and moved the family from the Philadelphia suburbs to Pittsburgh two years earlier. My older brother, Billy, was the only immediate family member still in the area. I called him and left a message.

My father-in-law came to see me and brought a red rose in a small crystal vase. He cried as he hugged me, saying, "I'm so sorry." I was touched by his visit and gift, but I was also beginning to feel angry. I knew we had serious problems to deal with, but nobody seemed to notice the good part—*I just had a baby!*

I did an ink sketch of the rose in the vase and fell asleep. Tad came back in the afternoon. Cody's back operation was successful; she was sleeping when he left. We would not be allowed to touch her, but we could see her through the glass in the morning.

Early the next day, Tad and I drove downtown to Thomas Jefferson University Hospital to see our daughter. Entering the neonatal intensive care unit nursery, I saw dozens of at-risk babies on the other side of a glass wall, each in a clear plastic drawer-like bed. This was a world I did not know existed. Some of the bandaged infants had undergone surgeries. Some were about to have surgery, like the baby born that morning with his heart on the outside of his chest. I watched the small heart, a living organ, beating in front of my eyes. *How was this possible?* A baby girl was born with her esophagus not connected to her stomach. Another infant with spina bifida had been abandoned in the unit right after his birth. His parents refused to take him home. I learned later that one of the nurses adopted him.

The suffering represented in this place astounded me. After twenty-two years without having anything close to a tragic experience, I now glimpsed a profound and sober reality. I imagined hospitals all across the country and throughout the world with intensive care nurseries full of babies like these. I was amazed I'd not known about them before. Now knowing, I was overcome with an emotion I could not describe—a feeling like gratitude. I felt honored to be a witness and share the ache and hope for these vulnerable infants.

I walked faster past each baby, looking for Cody. I'd seen her only for a few moments before she was taken away the day before. I hoped I'd recognize her. At the far end of the front row of plastic beds, I saw "Cody Jane" handwritten on tape on a plastic bed where she lay sleeping. A tiny diaper partially covered a bandage on her lower back. I wanted to touch her and feel her soft blonde hair again, but I could only watch her through the glass.

A neurosurgeon explained that Cody was born with the most severe type of spina bifida, called myelomeningocele. There was no indication of feeling or movement from her waist down; she might never have bowel or bladder control. No one could say if she would live, and no one knew what caused this birth defect or whether her brain was damaged.

He explained another, more serious, complication now that the exposed area at the lower end of Cody's spinal cord was surgically closed. There might be a corresponding open area at the top end of her spinal cord, inside her head. If so, cerebrospinal fluid could build up. Increased fluid pressure against her brain might cause permanent damage, seizures, and/or blindness. Cody's head would be measured each day for any sign of faster-than-normal growth.

Tad had graduated from Temple University the previous year and worked as a dishwasher while searching for a teaching job. Since my graduation from Moore College of Art three months earlier, we lived in Bucks County, assisting in a home renovation for my sculpture professor, Robert. We were thrilled when he invited us to move, with our two beagles and two cats, to the country for the few months before the birth of our baby. But now, staying in contact with Cody's doctors was our highest priority.

Tad and I drove the hour from Bucks Country to Philadelphia every other day. I spoke with specialists daily to track her progress and monitor her care. The glass wall continued to separate us from our newborn.

During a phone call with the pediatric resident, I was told Cody had "deformed" arms. Her arms had looked perfect to me. Alarmed, I drove into town to speak with the orthopedic surgeon, who assured me that Cody's arms were "entirely normal."

I asked, "Why did the pediatrician tell me that?"

The physician sighed and explained that doctors want to provide information so badly in "these types of cases" that they sometimes "see things that aren't there, or they make things up."

Incredulous, I asked, "Make things up?"

The doctor nodded and apologized for her less-experienced colleague.

Within three weeks the neurosurgeon confirmed that Cody's head was expanding more quickly than normal. He explained our options. He could implant a shunt in Cody's head. The one-way pump would route spinal fluid through tubing threaded into a vein to her heart. The fluid would absorb naturally into her bloodstream. The doctor said the shunt procedure was relatively new—successful for the first time about fifteen years earlier on a baby boy in Australia. Prior to that, infants like Cody usually died soon after birth.

As the doctor paused to write a note, I remembered singing with my high school choir at a nursing home with the gruesome name, The Inglis Home for Incurables. A man there in a reclining wheelchair had a head the size of a double-long football—too heavy for him to lift. We were told he had "water on the brain," or hydrocephalus.

Cody's doctor continued, "The other alternative is not to operate."

"And do what instead?" I asked, hoping for a less-invasive option.

Without expression, he answered, "Well, you could just wait. She might die."

Astonished, I asked, "Is that your recommendation?"

"No. But it's your choice."

I asked, "You said that without this operation our child will eventually become brain-damaged by fluid buildup, right?"

"Well, of course. If she lives," he clarified in a flat voice.

Annoyed, I said, "That's not a choice."

Cody was taken into surgery for the successful implantation of a shunt in her brain. Another baby born at that hospital around the same time required eleven shunt surgeries in eleven weeks.

For the next three weeks I pressed the doctors to let us take Cody home. We had moved to a small apartment north of downtown in a less-than-prosperous section of Germantown, and Tad had begun a teaching job in a school for "severely and profoundly retarded" adults.

The neurosurgeon agreed that Cody could come home if we could care for the gaping wound on her back. When I saw the incision for the first time, my tiny baby looked like she'd been sawn in half. The surgery to repair the opening on the lower end of her spine left a deep S-shaped open incision that curved from the right side of her waist down and through her left buttock. Dressing changes twice a day required a three-step cleansing and disinfecting process. Healing would take weeks, and the scar would be ugly.

Cody was also sent home with small plaster casts on her feet. She was born with a perfectly formed baby body except for her feet. Both were turned at the ankles as though swept to the left. The casts had to be changed weekly, then biweekly, then monthly for four months. After that, she'd wear a crossbar with shoes to hold her feet straight at night.

The day I held Cody for the first time since the morning of her birth, I touched her soft skin and inhaled her intoxicating baby scent. Watching her through the nursery glass for her first six weeks had been soundless. Tad and I laughed to hear her soft squeaks and coos. Her lips smacked as she sucked on her bottle. She made an audible sigh with each breath as she slept on the ride home.

I carried Cody in a bassinette from the car. Tad walked ahead to open the front door to our apartment. Cody was asleep on her tummy with her head turned to the left, her arms folded up on each side of her head, and her fingers closed in loose little fists. Her pale skin was almost transparent.

As I reached the steps to our door, I looked down at Cody. Her face was blue! She looked dead! I said an urgent prayer, "Please, God! Help!"

Cody's skin immediately returned to its pale color and, in the same second, she smiled in her sleep, a full cheek-dimpling smile. Instantly relieved, I thanked God. This was at once my first truly panicked moment of fear for Cody and immediate answer-to-prayer miracle.

I held Cody in my arms much of each day while Tad was at work. We kept busy with wound care, feedings, diaper changes, physical therapy exercises, kisses, and general entertainment. I tried to paint while Cody napped, but I had to stop before I could squeeze colors on the palette. Her naps were rare and short. I usually collapsed in exhaustion on the bed with her and the dogs.

Cody's first laugh erupted when our beagle, Mort, jumped onto the bed where Cody leaned on a pillow. He sat in front of her, tilted his head, and licked her cheek. Her cascade of deep chortles and squeaks repeated like a machine gun. I entertained her any way I could to see her eyes sparkle and hear that sound. Our dogs were guaranteed triggers for her amusement. Cody watched everything they did with rapt attention. She sometimes fell over laughing at them. Both beagles allowed her to pull their legs, tails, or ears as she reached for them. They licked her face, nuzzled her, and sometimes fell asleep in a pile together. With the dogs' help, Cody learned how to hold her head up without wobbling, roll over and, finally, sit up.

For the most part, I thought Cody wasn't so different from other babies. Other infants couldn't walk or control their bladders, either. An undeniable difference was that she saw lots of doctors: neurosurgeons, neurologists, urologists, orthopedic surgeons, pediatricians, wound care specialists, and a variety of physical therapists and adaptive equipment designers. She saw specialists at Jefferson Hospital and a highly recommended pediatrician for regular baby care.

The neurosurgeon was the most critical member of Cody's medical team. Shunt problems sounded the most life threatening. Tad and I were cautioned to watch for symptoms of a shunt malfunction. Possibilities included nausea, fatigue, headache, and the inability of her eyes to look up past the midpoint or horizon—a symptom called "sunsetting." The other symptoms could happen to anyone, so sunsetting eyes became the sign I watched for when Cody was ill.

Tad and I learned everything we could about each assault on Cody's health. Every new problem brought new treatment techniques. The medicines, procedures, and paraphernalia used to repair my child were both ghoulish and miraculous.

We studied alternative healing approaches to find anything else that might help Cody. Of special interest was information about how children with disabilities learn, and the types of experiences they often miss due to physical limitations—such as outdoor play. In the early spring, we took walks in an arboretum a few miles away. On the ground Cody wiggled forward on her elbows, played in the grass or leaned back on a resting beagle. Cody was nine months old when she spoke her first word: "dog."

When Cody awoke from a longer-than-usual nap one day in June, her eyes looked funny. I called Tad, and he came home early from work. He agreed that her eyes might be sunsetting. The pediatrician sent us to Children's Hospital of Pennsylvania (CHOP) in West Philadelphia.

Tad and I followed Cody's gurney from test to test. A CAT scan showed enlarged brain ventricles due to intracranial fluid buildup. Brain surgery to revise Cody's shunt was scheduled for the next morning. Tad left for the night and I stayed with Cody. I said silent prayers as she slept in a raised hospital crib in a large room with other cribs. The lights were low. Glass-enclosed rooms on one side were brightly lit where nurses worked on charts or spoke on the phone. I looked around at sleeping babies and was reminded of my first visit to an intensive care nursery. I was back in the company of others living through hard times.

A baby girl not much older than Cody sat in a crib nearby with her eyes open. She had a pretty face and dark hair, but the shape of her head was wrong. Her head hadn't developed above her eyebrows; she had no forehead. The next time a nurse walked by, I asked her to tell me about the little girl. The nurse said the child had been living at the hospital since birth and wasn't expected to survive this long. She'd been born with no actual brain, only a brainstem. She could open her eyes, sleep and breathe, but nothing beyond involuntary brain functions. That a child could look around, but have no thoughts, sounded like science fiction.

I sat in a chair next to Cody's crib and watched her sleep. In the early morning light, she opened her eyes, looked up at me and smiled. Her eyes were back to normal. I quickly called a nurse. I thanked God when the doctor examined Cody and cancelled surgery.

Before we left, a social worker told us about a new CHOP outpatient clinic for kids like Cody who needed care from multiple clinicians. The intent was to coordinate treatment by combined visits with several specialists in one monthly appointment—a sensible idea that could significantly reduce the frequency of doctor visits.

The following week, at the first appointment, the unsmiling pediatrician in charge of the clinic prescribed antibiotics for a urinary tract infection and directed that Cody take them on a permanent basis. When Tad and I questioned that, the doctor firmly stated that kidney infections were the most serious threat to Cody's health. Driving home her point, she added, "That's what *kills* these kids!"

Tad and I were instructed in the "Crede" technique. We were shown how to press on Cody's lower abdomen above the pubic bone to empty her bladder completely with each diaper change. The technique was intended to prevent buildup of bacteria in her urine that wouldn't fully flush out otherwise. The doctor said the harmless method wasn't uncomfortable. The first time I pressed down, I was afraid I might hurt Cody. But she didn't seem to mind.

Cody was eleven months old in mid-July when Tad's college roommate, Barry, invited us to his parents' home in New Hampshire for the weekend. He suggested a hike in the nearby White Mountains. A nature hike was the type of experience I'd read that kids with disabilities rarely have. As we drove north into New England, Cody laughed watching the dogs' ears flutter in the wind as they leaned out the car window.

When we arrived, Barry's father, a chiropractor, offered to examine Cody and x-ray her spine. He saw a twist in her pelvis and made an adjustment that successfully aligned her hips. As he lifted Cody from the padded table, her legs extended straighter. Her feet appeared to hang evenly together for the first time! Barry's father explained that with proper alignment of her spine, Cody might show improvement in other areas as well. He offered to identify a colleague in our area so Cody could continue the good progress when we returned to Philadelphia. This new development was exciting.

Barry had chosen Mount Jefferson for our hike the next morning. He and his fiancée Judy were experienced outdoor folks. They had canteens, cooking gear, rope, a large plastic tarp and tent, and maps of the trails. Barry assured us that the well-worn path up the mountain was easy going for novice hikers. We'd pitch the tent and sleep overnight on the summit of the second largest mountain in the Presidential Mountain Range.

As Barry described the distance we'd walk, I realized it wasn't a good idea to take both dogs with us after all. Sadie was a healthy two-year-old. But Morty, at age eleven, had arthritis in his hind leg. I didn't want to exacerbate his discomfort or risk injury. Barry's parents offered to keep Morty while we spent the night on the mountaintop.

Tad carried our supplies in a backpack, and Cody perched in a baby carrier on my back. I breathed in fresh mountain air as we started up the trail. The rhythm of my steps on the dirt path lulled Cody to sleep. The sun shone on the glossy black fur on Sadie's back. Her tail wagged in tempo as the six of us made our way up the mountain.

The trail had been on a winding but steady incline for more than an hour when we discovered that none of us had filled our canteens. Barry pulled out the map and suggested an alternative trail that wound sideways to the closest water source. We agreed we'd gone too far to go back down the mountain, so we set out for the stream. Cody slept during the long detour.

Our path crossed some loose rock on a steep slant. I stepped out onto the scree, lost my footing, and felt sheer panic for the split second it took to grab a tree branch and regain balance. In that brief instant, I pictured Cody tumbling out of the back carrier and down the mountain. I cringed to realize I'd put her at such risk. *What was I thinking to bring her up here?*

Too late to turn back, our only option was to keep moving toward drinking water. Tad and I switched packs. I carried the heavier supply pack; he carried our precious cargo. I walked close behind and kept my eye on Cody as the adrenalin coursing through my body slowly dissipated. Sadie never lost her footing and trotted on without hesitation.

The sun was directly overhead when we reached the stream. Sadie put her paws in the sparkling cold water and took a long drink. I filled a bottle for Cody, gulped water by the handful, and filled canteens. We sat down and pulled out snacks. Barry unfolded the trail map to plot our next move. Reaching the summit before evening wasn't a realistic expectation in light of our detour. He recommended heading for the emergency shelter for the night.

After another hour on the trail, we came to a wooden sign with a warning: *Set up camp before dark or turn back! People have been known to die of exposure on this mountain even in the summertime.* That sounded ominous, but the afternoon sun felt warm. We decided to step up our pace. The steepness of the less-traveled path looked like more than Sadie could maneuver at points, but she plodded onward and upward.

Our progress was a little slower when the sun moved past the top of the mountain, leaving us in shadow and imminent darkness. None of us expected such an abrupt change. We continued on until, without warning, it began to rain. Looking up, it was clear that going forward required using rope to pull us over the next ledge. Our hiking party was stuck on a slanted area about six-by-six-feet square. Fat raindrops splashed us, and thunder began. There was no time to set up camp. Barry pulled out the plastic tarp and we scurried to stretch out underneath before the ground was drenched. Our only choice was to stay put, do without dinner, and try to sleep until daybreak.

The four of us lay side by side. Cody lay quietly on my stomach. Sadie cuddled between Tad and me. Barry was closest to the outside ledge. He suggested we tuck our hiking boots under our right sides to prevent rolling over the edge in our sleep.

Cold rain battered the plastic tarp. Lightning flashed to our side and down the mountain. I hoped the thunder and drumming rain muffled my voice when I whispered to Tad that I was scared. He turned and put his arm over Cody and me. Tears slid down the sides of my face. I was truly terrified. I couldn't tell if Barry or Judy slept, but they were silent through the night.

The storm carried on for several hours. Cody's diaper was saturated; my denim shirt was soaked with warm pee. But I could not move to change her. Safety lay in holding still and trying to sleep. I saw an occasional flash of lightning reflected in my daughter's trusting eyes as she looked up toward my face. I prayed for God to rescue us, to bring us safely off this mountain. I wanted to be way below in any of the tiny houses I knew were down there from the twinkling lights I'd seen in the distance before the downpour. I was glad Morty was spared this experience. I imagined him safe, dry, and curled up asleep.

The rain stopped sometime in the night. The moment it was light, we climbed out from under the tarp and folded it into a pack. The sky was blue and cloudless—the start of a gorgeous sunny day. Barry used the rope to climb up over the ledge, where he discovered that we were above the tree line. He came back down for Sadie, tucked her under his left arm and pulled them both to higher ground with his right arm.

Tad secured Cody in the backpack and he, Judy, and I climbed up over the ledge. Once on open tundra, Barry used twigs to coax a campfire. Within minutes, a park ranger appeared wearing shorts, hiking boots and a wide-brimmed hat. He said fires weren't allowed in the protected tundra. He kicked dirt onto the still-tiny flames, explaining that flora on the tundra was so fragile that a campfire could destroy what took thousands of years to grow. As the ranger pointed to miniature plants, moss, and flowers growing between the rocks, I coveted his clean khaki shirt. While he wrote a ticket and attached a hefty fine, I thought, *Where was this guy last night when I thought we might die on the mountain?* Out loud I said, "We were stuck on a ledge all night during the thunderstorm."

"You were lucky, ma'am." He folded the citation and handed it to Barry. "Three people fell down the ravine in the past week; they all died."

Yikes.

The ranger left as quickly as he had appeared and we repacked our supplies. Since Cody's food was in small jars and Sadie's dry food was in a plastic bag, they were the only ones who ate that morning. As I spooned applesauce into Cody's mouth, her lips smacked, and I pondered the danger we'd survived. *That could have easily been us tumbling down a ravine.*

Once packed up, we looked around at the field of boulders between our current location on the craggy tundra and trail markings that resumed in the distance. Between the large rocks were wide gaps and deep fissures. With no indication which direction led to the trail, we each attempted different routes and repeatedly met with crevasses too wide to cross. The giant rocky maze stopped us at every turn. Dear little Sadie solved our dilemma and earned respect from our seasoned hiking friends. She wound methodically across the broad expanse, leading us back onto the trail. We never did see the emergency shelter.

When our hiking party arrived at the mountain's summit, at an elevation of more than 5,700 feet, we marveled at a view that went for miles into the distance. I lifted Cody out of the back carrier and pointed to the far-off horizon in several directions. She looked with interest everywhere I pointed and seemed to agree it was special.

After our night on the ledge, we chose not to linger any longer than it took to eat a quick meal and pack up. The five-mile direct descent went fast. Once at the bottom, I looked back up at magnificent Mount Jefferson. I cringed again to think I'd taken a baby and a dog up there and clung to a ledge for hours amid booming thunder and lightning. But we'd escaped unharmed and the sun had shone brightly in the morning. Our small dog had turned out to be an essential member of our hiking team. Perhaps without the detour to find drinking water, our trek would not have been so precarious; but I'd never forget how vulnerable I felt and how frightened I was for my precious family that night on the ledge.

Chapter 2

Toddling

ONCE BACK IN THE CITY, I put renewed effort into Cody's exercise regimen and we celebrated her first birthday. During our next CHOP clinic appointment, I told the physical therapist that a chiropractor had adjusted Cody's hips so her legs extended evenly for the first time. I explained how prior to that, Cody's right leg extended lower than her left leg due to a hip rotation. Using Barry's father's words, I went on, "By repeating an adjustment of Cody's right ilium, the corrective result might eventually become permanent and possibly improve her residual nerve function."

My excitement in sharing this information was met with a frown on the face of the clinician. "Are you saying you intend to allow a chiropractor to treat your daughter?"

I explained that the chiropractor in New Hampshire conducted an extensive evaluation that included x-rays. He'd sent his findings and films to the Gonstead Clinic of Chiropractic in Wisconsin and received confirmation of his assessment. But a consultation had not yet been scheduled with a chiropractor in our area.

"Well," she responded, "if you plan to see another chiropractor, even for a consultation, you cannot continue to bring Cody here."

When I asked why, the clinician said, "Splintering of services is against clinic policy." She said we had to make a choice: "See a chiropractor, or continue to come to Children's."

I was stupefied. I asked, "If you had a child like Cody, wouldn't you do anything to help her? Wouldn't you try anything that might work?"

"I see your point, but you still have to choose."

Several other parents stood nearby listening to our conversation. One mother followed us to the door and in a hushed voice said, "My son's being treated by a chiropractor, too. It's making a difference. His spine was twisted and now it's straight. I just don't tell them here."

Tad and I chose to return Cody to the outpatient care of individual physicians at Thomas Jefferson University Hospital. Just in case, we never mentioned the chiropractic care that we continued to find helpful.

Later that fall, I began working Fridays at a suburban mental health clinic near the school where Tad taught. The three of us drove to work together. Cody spent the day with Tad while I typed, filed, and helped with patients in the clinic. She often spent Friday nights with Tad's parents.

After Tad and I considered potential limits on education that Cody might face, he enrolled in a graduate program in special education so he'd be qualified to homeschool her if conventional schooling wasn't available. The advanced degree led to his becoming director of the school for severely and profoundly retarded adults.

A move to a small house in the western suburb of Paoli brought Tad and me closer to our jobs. To help with the mounting expense of graduate school, and healthcare costs not covered by medical insurance, Tad took a temporary job loading food trucks before work in the morning. I worked more days at the mental health clinic as my responsibilities increased. As time and Cody allowed, I did some freelance painting and illustration.

Before going to our regular jobs each day, we dropped Cody at a nearby county daycare program for "special needs" kids. Tad had classes four nights a week. We soldiered on, juggling work, school, Cody's care and her medical needs, without acknowledging the strain that threatened to overwhelm us.

Despite our mounting stress, Cody was a cheerful toddler, even though she couldn't toddle. She was talkative and enjoyed throwing kisses with her hands. She moved her shoulders with the beat of music and enjoyed games with hand movements. *Hawaii Five-O* was her favorite television show; she liked scenes with people talking on telephones. Holding a telephone, throwing kisses, and raising both hands in the air at the same time were some of the exercises that helped her develop balance and strengthen her upper body. Cody scurried about on a wheelie toy she stretched out on and pulled herself around with her arms.

We placed her crib mattress on top of milk crates against our bedroom wall with a padded board slanted from the bed to the floor so Cody could safely scoot out of bed on her tummy. If Tad and I slept later on weekends, she was happy to lie in bed and sing, or crawl out of bed and play on the floor.

A few months before Cody's second birthday, Tad and I received an invitation from the Pediatric Society of Jefferson Medical School to be a part of an informal discussion with professors, medical students, and parents of children with birth defects. The goal was an interchange to help future pediatricians go "beyond the textbook" to educate and acquaint themselves with the "dilemmas, hardships, joys, and realities" of treating children with disabilities. The letter noted that frequently the pediatrician is of little help to the parents, and only the parent of such a child can communicate the impact of the situation. The gathering was the brainchild of Dr. Gary Carpenter in the pediatrics department. I admired him already for the care he'd directed for Cody, and felt another kinship in that he was a watercolor painter.

Since Cody's birth, we'd dealt with plenty of medical professionals. Tad and I found it refreshing to be asked for *our* opinions. We agreed to participate.

Twenty-four people sat around a large conference table in the Alumnae Hall at the medical school on a Wednesday evening. Introductions were made and the goal was restated. Medical students and physicians were to listen. Parents were asked to describe life with their children.

One seven-year-old required medication that only partially controlled grand mal seizures that occurred several times each day. He wore a helmet to protect his head during seizures. He might collapse anywhere for several minutes, his arms and legs flailing. Sometimes he bit his tongue. This family was on constant alert.

Another family had a child with "severe mental retardation." She couldn't speak or care for herself and would have abilities of an infant all her life. Some of Tad's students were the adult versions of this child. The parents worried about their daughter's future. Who would care for her after they died?

A mother described her twelve-year-old son who was born blind and without legs. I found myself feeling grateful that Cody could see and speak. The more these parents spoke, the more grateful I felt.

After hearing from each family, including our own story, group members shared their reactions. Physicians expressed gratitude for the valuable information; medical students expressed awe at the magnitude of responsibility shouldered by the parents. Every parent felt the way I did. We were grateful to have our own circumstances instead of any of those others.

The mother of the child with the seizure disorder said, "I'm so glad my child can walk. I can't imagine how hard his life would be in a wheelchair."

I thought, at least Cody *has* legs; she can see, hear, talk, and laugh. I don't have to worry when she's out of my sight that she might collapse and swallow her tongue.

Dr. Carpenter summarized the view that clinicians must respect and listen to parents, the true experts who care for their kids day to day. Parents know their own children far better than a doctor who meets them for arranged appointments or during hospital emergencies. He said to never forget this. I left the gathering feeling validated, respected—and wishing all physicians were like Dr. Carpenter.

That fall, Cody needed a "hip and knee release" operation to loosen tendons to straighten her legs so she could wear long-leg braces. For normal leg bone growth, Cody needed to bear weight in a standing posi-tion. She'd be in a full-length body cast for six weeks after surgery. While in the cast, she couldn't attend the daycare program with her friends. Unable to pay for outside help or risk losing either of our jobs, Tad and I felt enormous relief when my mother came from Pittsburgh to help out.

She had seen Cody only twice and still hesitated before touching her. Presuming that Cody was fragile, Mom was afraid of hurting her. Six weeks in each other's company changed that. Cody was full of energy despite the restriction of a body cast. With the back down on her stroller she could lie on her stomach and prop herself up on her elbows during long walks. My mother read aloud, sang, and played games with Cody. Mom saw that Cody was a strong and active two-year-old who laughed and loved easily.

Over the next year, Cody attended her daycare program and Tad finished his master's degree. I finished postgraduate psychology courses and became a caseworker at the clinic. We scrimped to pay off the school loans and planted a garden to save money on food.

Cody grew stronger. Her shoulders and arms were sturdy from dragging the weight of her paralyzed lower body as she crawled. She lingered in the hallway at the top of the staircase and wanted to follow Mort and Sadie down the carpeted steps. I sat in front of her as she moved forward on her tummy and lowered her body from step to step. I showed her how to stay close to the balusters and grab one if needed to steady herself. She was enthusiastic in her attempts. We practiced together until she could reach the bottom of the stairs without help.

Both dogs paid close attention to her movements. Like a bodyguard and protector, Mort had always positioned himself between Cody and any guests who entered our home. When he became ill and died the same month a car ran over our youngest cat, I had the difficult task of explaining death to a three-year-old.

Chapter 3

Big House, Big Wheels, Big Surgery

I WAS FAMILIAR with the literature that gave poor odds on the success of a marriage when there is a "special needs" child. However, I didn't take the dismal prediction seriously. Only in retrospect could I see how fears and strains associated with Cody may have affected Tad and me. I loved Tad, admired his passion for poetry and music, and shared his interest in spiritual enlightenment and a life of purpose. But on several occasions he made dramatic life changes to follow his conscience and perceived destiny, which ultimately led away from me.

Though I had imagined myself with Tad forever, the marriage aspect of our relationship unraveled during this period. We decided we were better suited as best friends and co-parents. Finally acknowledging the strain we had been under, we took a practical approach to finding a solution to our isolation and stress. A friend told us about a seven-bedroom house for rent in the suburb of Bryn Mawr. A big house shared with others might provide a larger community of supportive friendship. By adding four other housemates, we could each have a room, with an extra room on the first floor for a painting studio.

A possible housemate was a friend Tad and I met at a party at the University of Pennsylvania. Dennis was a tall, slender Australian with sandy-colored hair and a ginger beard. He came to Penn on a Fulbright scholarship to obtain a Ph.D. in economics. He hated living in a university dorm in the city, so he jumped at the invitation to our house in Paoli and brought an English friend.

In January, a month before our move to the big house, Dennis and Ian arrived for the weekend. I called out to Cody to come downstairs and meet our guests. She'd mastered the method of descending the carpeted staircase on her belly like an alligator. She did it so fast she sometimes alarmed people who thought she was falling down the stairs.

Cody loved to meet new people. She rushed to the bottom of the staircase, gave our friends a wide smile, raised her fist, and declared, "Baby Power!"

Our guests were charmed.

Later that evening, Dennis asked more about Cody. He wanted to know why she couldn't walk. I described her congenital birth defect, back surgery, and shunt. Most people I met had not heard of spina bifida or shunts, but Dennis nodded along as I talked about Cody. I told him the shunt was a relatively new invention—used successfully for the first time on a boy in Australia. Dennis nodded again. "Right, that was my brother."

"Are you kidding?"

Dennis assured me that his brother Mark was the first child in the world to survive with a shunt, and offered to show me the Australian newspaper clippings. Mark was born with hydrocephalus, resulting in slight brain damage. Now a teenager, he still had the same shunt.

Astounded, I felt shivers on my arms and up and down my spine— the feeling I later came to think of as angel shivers.

Dennis and Ian became our new housemates, along with Tad's brother Teddy and my work friend, Valerie. Tad, Valerie, Cody, and I had bedrooms on the second floor of the big house. Teddy, Dennis, and Ian had third-floor rooms. Cody spun around in her hand-controlled wheelie toys as the housemates worked together to paint each room. "Family" meetings were initiated to plan shared meals, assign chores, and address any problems. The best part of our group-living experiment was that there were more people around to interact with Cody. Tad played his guitar and our housemates often joined in as we sang her to sleep at night. One friend after another carried Cody around at our housewarming party. She laughed, made silly jokes, and enjoyed the attention.

Though Tad and I no longer lived as a couple, we were in no rush to divorce. He developed new friendships that didn't involve me and published a book of poetry. I worked mornings and took classes. Cody attended a preschool program for children with disabilities.

During the summer my mornings were free until Cody's day camp started at 11:00 a.m. Her morning bath was in the old-fashioned deep kitchen sink where she balanced more safely than in a tub.

Most days, I sketched Cody and we chatted while she stood strapped in her leg braces. On sunny days she sat on the ground outside, picked peapods, and played with Sadie while I weeded the garden. I dropped Cody at camp on my way to work. Tad picked her up from camp, and she spent the last part of the day at his school. Some of his students were more childlike than Cody, and she was drawn to their sweetness.

One afternoon Cody saw a student become upset and slap his own head several times and pull his hair. To stop the behavior, Tad took Ronnie to a room away from others until he calmed down. That evening, when Cody became angry about something, she copied Ronnie's behavior and slapped her own head. I said in a firm voice, "Cody, it's not okay to hit yourself."

She stopped. But at breakfast the next morning when I said no to her request for another cracker, she started to cry and pull her hair. I warned, "If you are going to do that, you're going to be treated the same way Ronnie was." I picked her up, carried her into the living room, and left to go back to the kitchen.

Cody screamed, "No, Mommy!"

I asked, "Will you calm down?" She said yes and surprised me by becoming calm instantly. Back in the kitchen, she resumed playing and chattered while I rinsed breakfast dishes.

By the time Cody turned four in August, she learned to ride around the house in her first wheelchair. She adapted with ease to greater mobility and independence. She maneuvered through the downstairs with increasing speed in her heavy Everest Jennings chair. She learned how to avoid bumping into furniture or pinching her fingers in doorways. She was fitted with new leg braces, but had little interest in trying to walk with them. A welder friend made a set of parallel bars that we kept on the front porch. Standing practice required effort on all our parts. Cody would not be forced. She now cried whenever I strapped the metal and plastic forms around her pelvis, legs, and feet. She said she felt scared standing up between the bars; she was afraid of falling. Her therapists tried to teach her how to fall safely, but that further terrified her. The only way to log standing time was if someone held her. Even then she was miserable. I gave in too often. Tad thought I should be tougher about it, but it broke my heart to see her cry so despondently. The process became the source of many arguments between Tad, Cody, and me.

During our first six months in the big house, I spent increasing time with Dennis. I found his Australian accent exotic and his droll sense of humor entertaining. He taught me about jazz and economics. He loaned me his copy of Virginia Woolf's *A Room of One's Own*; I was impressed that he'd underlined many passages. I began to imagine the camaraderie of our household as akin to the writers, artists, and economists of London's Bloomsbury Group in the 1920s and '30s. Dennis had bags of cameras and lenses and took some of the best photographs ever of Cody. His affection for her was obvious, and she adored him. She liked to ride high in a backpack when he took her on walks. He showed her how to play records and tapes, and how to use a headset so she could listen to her own music in the same room while I sketched and he studied. Dennis joined us every night in Cody's room at bedtime for goodnight kisses and songs.

A string of troubles began that fall with a visit to the student clinic at Penn. After watching a nurse take a blood sample, Dennis fainted as we left the clinic. He revived quickly and I learned it wasn't the first time he "passed out," as Dennis preferred to describe it.

Tad moved out of the house after a disagreement with another housemate. I told him, "This is weird. You had a problem with someone else, but you moved away from Cody and me, too. Do you think it's time for us to get that divorce?" Tad agreed. It was weird, and divorce finally did make sense. He explained to Cody that he'd still see her every day, but sleep at his parents' house. I hoped she'd adjust to the change the way she seemed to easily adapt to whatever happened. But Cody cried for Tad every night at bedtime.

I drove her to preschool each day and picked her up from Tad's school on my way home from work. One drizzly October morning after dropping Cody at school, a tow truck ran a light and smashed into my car. The driver-side window broke over my head, filling my mouth with glass, and my body with pain. My car was demolished. Due to a concussion, sprained neck, gashes on my head, shoulder, and hand, I was instructed by the emergency room doctor not to lift my child for three months. *Right.*

For several days, Cody and Sadie played or dozed on my bed while I leaned back on pillows with my neck in a brace. I made it though the next few painful weeks with help from Dennis and prescription pain-killers. Valerie drove me to and from work, where I shut my office door and lay on the floor for several minutes between patient appointments. Cody and I sat together each evening on my bed as I recovered from the day. She entertained visitors, told stories, and directed friends to sing for me, telling us all to hold hands. She made everyone laugh even if her jokes didn't make sense.

Cody had regular clinic appointments and no bus to preschool, so a car was a necessity. My brother Charlie offered me his old car for a hundred dollars. My parents drove the car from Charlie's home in St. Louis and spent part of the Christmas holiday with us in the big house.

Learning that Dennis was now more than a friend, my father immediately asked to speak with him in private. Dennis looked nervous following Dad into the kitchen. But once alone, Dad asked him to persuade me to have an operation I'd been avoiding. One of the infamous Dalcon Shield birth control devices had punctured my uterus a few years before and become lodged somewhere in my pelvic region. My doctor had firmly recommended its removal, saying it entailed only a "simple side slash." Dad had been pressing me to have the operation ever since. Dennis readily promised my compliance.

I dreaded feeling incapacitated again. I needed full strength to care for Cody. However, I had the operation in January. Only days later, a fire destroyed the clinic where I worked. Staff met in a temporary space, trying to recover patient care information from drenched paper files. Tad dropped by the office space a week before Valentine's Day to report that our divorce was final. We went out to lunch to toast the future.

The final and largest bead on the string of troubles occurred on Valentine's Day. Cody woke up glassy-eyed, complaining of a bad headache. When I prompted her to look up, she couldn't. Her eyes were sunsetting. I phoned the doctor, described Cody's eyes, and was told to bring her to the emergency department at CHOP.

Cody held still while she was x-rayed, making only a few pitiful sobs near the end as her head pain increased. After the scanning procedure, she was groggy and fell asleep. Dennis waited with Cody and me in the emergency room cubicle.

The neurosurgeon who spoke with us was a Scottish man in a well-tailored suit and cowboy boots. His warm manner was not typical for a neurosurgeon in my experience up until then, or (to be candid) for most of Cody's life. He said the x-ray showed that the shunt tubing no longer reached Cody's heart, and there was a blockage. His plan was to route a new shunt to her abdominal cavity instead of her heart.

Dennis and I followed as Cody was taken to a hospital room. The doctor and nurses who checked on her could barely rouse her. She awoke only as she was transferred to a rolling gurney. I explained to Cody that the doctor was going to fix her headache and that she was on the way to the operating room. She grabbed my hand and wouldn't release me even to let me walk around the gurney.

I tried to make her laugh by making faces as if I were being crushed when we squeezed through the doorway of her room. She laughed and let me come around to the other side. Dennis and I each held one of her hands as she was rolled down the hall. At the double doors to the operating room, Cody tightened her grip and said, "I don't want to go in."

"Are you worried?" I asked in my most soothing mom voice.

She whimpered, "Yes, I am."

I assured her, "You don't have to worry, sweetie. This operation is going to take away your bad headache. We'll be right here, waiting for you outside this door."

I leaned close and said a prayer for God to take care of Cody and keep her safe. I kissed her scared little face, and she was rolled through the doors.

Dennis and I waited in the "hospitality" room across the hall. Dr. Bruce said the procedure would take only thirty minutes, after which he'd come straight to us. Three hours later, with still no word, I was afraid that something went wrong. Tad left work and headed for the hospital. My stomach churned. After four hours, a nurse came out to explain that the operation started late. That was some relief. Finally, Dr. Bruce came to tell us that the operation went well and, as long as no fever or infection developed, Cody could go home in two days.

As her gurney was wheeled out of the recovery room, Cody looked like a wounded bird, with her arm taped to a board that held an IV in place. Part of her head was shaved and she had bandages on her head, neck, and stomach. I took her hand and kissed her sleepy face. In a quivering little voice, she said, "It wasn't so bad."

I was surging with love for my girl, grateful, and full of admiration for her resilience. I had feared the possibility of this operation for four years. Cody had faced the entire ordeal like a trooper with far more bravery than I could muster. I prayed this was her last shunt operation.

Once Cody was back in her hospital bed, I adjusted the covers and pillows to make her comfortable. She made a loud raspy, throat-grumbling sound. I must have had a horrified look on my face because she stopped and said, "I'm sorry, Mom. I had to do that."

As I helped her eat a Popsicle and sip ginger ale, Cody asked me to help her get rid of the IV in her arm. I told her it was just like the one I had for my operation a few weeks before. Cody looked up and asked, "You had one just like it?"

After I said yes, she didn't complain about it again.

Cody's roommate for the next two days was an eight-year-old named Laura. Several times a day, respiratory therapists performed a procedure that looked brutal at first. Laura lay on her stomach, and then on each side, while therapists slapped her back repeatedly with cupped hands. Laura had cystic fibrosis and the hollow slaps helped loosen lung secretions and made her cough. Sometimes a clear mask with moist air and medication was put over her nose and mouth to help her breathe. A nurse told me that Laura was not likely to live beyond her teenage years.

Like many hospital roommates Cody came to know with complex and painful medical problems, Laura behaved more like a mature adult than a child. I was impressed with her knowledge and matter-of-fact approach to her illness. She knew the names of medications and equipment; she worked with her nurses, followed directions, and gave a few.

Cody came home from the hospital with a chest cold. She asked for "one of those glass things to help me breathe," referring to Laura's nebulizer mask.

I was coaxing Cody to sleep on my bed when Sadie ran into the room, took a flying leap and landed in front of Cody's face. Our sweet beagle had been neglected for a few days. With a delighted smile, Cody said in a stuffed-up voice, "That was great, Mom. Sadie jumped up here all by herself."

As Cody fell asleep, I thought about all that had happened in recent months. Our year in the big house had started out as an exciting new adventure. But the last five months had been a steady string of crises. None of the drama and calamity compared to Cody's ordeal. As I watched her sleep with her arm on Sadie's belly, I thanked God that my four-year-old girl had survived her scary brain surgery. It was the first she would remember.

Chapter 4

Questions

AT A MARCH CLINIC APPOINTMENT, I was told to give Cody a suppository each evening to develop a habit of emptying her bowels at the same time each day. Like any kid, she hated holding still. And, no matter how well placed, the suppositories popped out unless she held still. The product never achieved the desired result, but we tried it for a while.

Tad came to help Cody in her leg braces one day in April. It was the usual struggle. She hadn't stood in braces since before her surgery. She was cranky and uncooperative. That evening as she lay on my bed, trying to be still, Cody began to cry. "Daddy's mad at me."

She was inconsolable. I phoned Tad and he tried to comfort her with loving words. But after saying goodbye, Cody thrust the phone at me, buried her head in a pillow, and sobbed. I called Tad again. He promised to come after school the next day to play. I cradled Cody in my arms that night until she fell asleep.

The next morning, she refused to wear shorts, saying, "I hate my legs," and, "My legs aren't pretty." She pulled her dress down to cover her knees. "Why can't I wear long pants all the time like you do?"

I told her she could wear long pants. "But I think your legs are pretty."

She frowned and said, "You're wrong."

Despite fun with Tad that day, Cody's demeanor was sober that evening as she held still on my bed. I suspected she was again thinking about her legs. I prompted her to talk.

"Babe, I don't want you to hate your legs. You have wonderful legs.

Do you think the reason you hate your legs is because they don't work the way they should?"

Cody lowered her eyes and said, "Yes. That's the reason."

I kissed each of her legs and said, "Your legs can't help it. I think we should decide to like your legs."

Cody thought a moment before saying, "Okay."

She switched topics: "I don't have any friends of my own." She named her babysitter Erica and said, "That's all the friends I have."

I reminded her of our many friends who loved her, but she protested, "None of them are just *my* friends."

When I said, "You're *my* best friend," her face lit up and she hugged me.

Hearing Dennis come downstairs from his third-floor room, Cody called out for him to please bring her a drink. Dennis yelled back from the hallway, "It's late. You've had enough to drink. No more tonight."

She took a deep breath, put her head down on her pillow, released a big sigh and said, "He's a shit."

I laughed out loud, and Cody glanced up at me and smiled.

The next day while she played on the floor in my room, I heard Cody say, "I like myself, but what's wrong with me?" When I asked what she meant, she said, "I was talking to myself!"

Later that same week she asked Dennis if it was okay for her to call him Daddy. He was touched and readily agreed. Cody happily told Tad, "I have two daddies now."

Tad hugged her and said she was lucky to have two dads. He had noticed Dennis's father-potential the previous summer during a visit with family friends before Cody had a wheelchair. Two visiting little girls ran through the house, excluding Cody from their play. After several minutes of trying to crawl after them, she began to cry in heartbreaking, pitiful sobs. I wasn't present when one of the girls pointed at Cody and said, "Your legs don't work, and you'll never walk by yourself."

Tad and Dennis had spun toward the little girl in unison and growled, "Shut up!"

On the Thursday before Easter, Tad and I took Cody to a clinic appointment. She was prescribed new leg braces, further appointments and tests were scheduled, and additional daily tasks were recommended. The urologist said the Crede technique we used for years to empty Cody's bladder was no longer considered a desirable practice. Pressing down on the bladder could force urine up the tiny ureter tubes and damage her kidneys. Instead, we were trained to catheterize Cody by inserting a short, lubricated stainless-steel tube into her urethra to drain urine every four hours.

She needed a test called an IVP, new antibiotics to prevent urinary tract infections, and more trips into town on workdays for the leg brace fittings. Each appointment meant two hours in traffic, and some of the catheter and sterilizing equipment was only available at a hard-to-find medical supply store. Cody missed the Easter party at school and I missed an important staff meeting at work. As I thought about all this on the ride home, tears slid down my face. Similarly somber, Tad reassured me. "You take care of the routine things. I'll make the trips and pick up the equipment and medication."

Oblivious to our concerns, Cody was laughing in the backseat about something funny the dog did that morning. Thinking how naturally she adjusted to inconvenience with cheerfulness and humor, I had to smile.

As summer approached, the owner of our big house decided to sell the property. Dennis, Cody, and I moved to an apartment. Sadie came with us. Our cat Emmy went to live with Tad.

While Cody was away at a seashore clinic camp in July, Dennis suggested marriage. I reminded him that he'd once said he'd never marry. He countered with a list of advantages: we loved each other, he loved Cody, he'd get a teaching job when he finished his Ph.D., and I could finish my master's degree tuition-free as the spouse of a professor.

His proposal was "practical" and we continued to talk about it. I knew Cody loved Dennis and he loved her. I often thought he preferred Cody's company to mine. I teased that he wanted to marry me so he could be her dad.

I consulted with Cody. "Do you think I should marry Dennis?"

She answered in a sincere tone, "I don't like that idea."

I asked why not, and she said, "Because I'd like to marry him myself."

Smiling, I explained that Dennis would be pretty old by the time she was old enough to get married. Cody thought that was a good point and said "in that case" it was okay for me to marry him.

Soon after turning five and starting kindergarten, Cody heard exciting news that she had a new cousin. Tad's sister Becky had married my former art teacher, Robert. We drove to Bucks County in early October to see the baby. After meeting her baby cousin, Cody asked new questions such as, "How does a mommy's body make milk?" Some questions were more difficult for me to answer, like, "Where does hair come from?" Her curiosity progressed to how God made people, why her legs didn't work, and what her shunt did. Several times, she said, "I'll be able to walk when I'm bigger."

I didn't know what to say to that. I wondered if Cody had some preternatural awareness of a coming miracle. Or, was she under the impression that her ability to walk was merely late in coming? I didn't want to squelch her faith, but I wanted her to have accurate information.

She asked me, "Why can you walk and I can't?"

I explained that her nerves didn't grow the way they were meant to and didn't connect properly for her legs to receive messages from her brain. "And I don't know why," I finally said.

I showed Cody that if I touched her arm, she could feel it, and she could make her arm move. I touched her leg to illustrate the difference. She saw that she couldn't feel my touch or make her leg move. Cody repeated, "But why can *you* walk?'

"That same problem didn't happen to me."

Cody changed the subject abruptly. "All my friends are pretend."

Conversation about legs had again turned to a discussion about friends.

At a recent party, Cody had behaved like an emcee-style hostess. She instructed guests to dance or sing and kept everyone laughing. She blossomed with personality around adults, but her teacher told me that Cody was shy around the other children in kindergarten.

I wasn't sure how to enlarge her friendship circle. Few of our friends had kids, and we didn't live near other children. I decided to take afternoons off work whenever I could so a school friend could come over to play with Cody.

On Halloween, Cody wore makeup and dressed as a gaucho in long pants, a straw hat, and a woolen poncho. Dennis said Halloween wasn't such a big deal in Australia when he was little, but with Cody he participated enthusiastically. He wheeled her across numerous bumpy lawns, pulled her up dozens of steps, and coached her about which candies to pick.

At age five, Cody's favorite singers were Barry Manilow, Dolly Parton, and Debbie Boone. She had memorized the lyrics to "You Light Up My Life" and sang along with the record. After three consecutive days of her begging to see Debbie Boone in person, I was convinced it wasn't just a passing interest. Dennis and I took her to a Debbie Boone concert.

Cody decided, "I want to be a singer when I grow up." She played with a tape recorder and sang into the microphone. On one recording she pretended to be Debbie Boone, and we carried on an interview:

"Ladies and Gentlemen," I said, "we are honored today to have the very famous, beautiful, and talented Debbie Boone with us. Welcome, Miss Boone."

Cody responded, "Please, call me Debbie."

"Thank you so much, Miss Boone, I am such a big fan!"

"Call me Debbie!"

"Yes, yes, Debbie. Will you please sing a song for your fans?"

"Yes, I will. It's called, 'You Light Up My Life.'"

Cody sang each verse, and when she finished, I said, "Oh, Miss Boone, you are such a talented and wonderful singer!"

"I said, call me Debbie!!"

"Of course, I'm sorry. Perhaps I can ask you another question. Are you familiar with the wonderful singer, Cody Cornell?"

Cody answered, "I do know her, yes."

"I just think she is so talented and wonderful, just like you, Miss Boone."

"Call me Debbie!!!"

"Okay, Debbie. Will you sing another song for us, please?"

"I only know 'You Light Up My Life.' That's the only song I know."

I had to interview Cody as Dolly Parton to hear a different song.

Christmas Eves were spent with Tad's family. He was the oldest of six, and his family sang Christmas carols together in blended harmonies like Von Trapps in *The Sound of Music*. The previous year, when Cody was four, she unwrapped dozens of toys and books and was saturated with festivity and cranky with exhaustion by the time she fell asleep. Only a few gifts were under our tree at home on Christmas morning. I'd sewn a doll and a dog, bought a few toys, and wrapped a bunch of bananas in tissue paper. Cody's eyes had shown the brightest when she tore open the tissue paper and, seeing her favorite fruit, shouted, "Bananas!"

On this Christmas Eve, her mature sincerity pierced me with sweetness as she stopped to thank the giver before opening each of her gifts.

Dennis, Cody, and I flew to Pittsburgh on Christmas day to visit my parents. That evening, we all sat around the fireplace. Cody was on one end of the couch. My father sat on the other end with his crossed legs resting on the coffee table. Cody scooted close to Dad, looked up and said, "Hello."

Deaf in one ear, my father didn't respond. Cody turned to me and said, "I think he's shy."

Hearing that, Dad smiled. Cody leaned close, kissed Dad, and hugged his arm. She spoke to him soothingly and called him Gordon, instead of Grandpa—or Peepaw, as she called Tad's father. She cajoled, teased, and tickled my father all evening, and he smiled at her attention. When we headed up to bed, Dad apologized to me for being "standoffish" with Cody. He said he didn't want her to catch his cold. But Cody was right. Dad *was* shy.

The next day, Cody stayed with Mom while Dad, Dennis, and I picked up groceries. Upon returning to the house, I took Cody to the bedroom to be cathed. She wore incontinent briefs in case of leakage between catheterizations. She didn't want anyone to refer to the briefs as "diapers." "Diapers are for babies." Cody was a "big kid," not a baby. So we called incontinent briefs "ibs," for short.

As I taped the sides of Cody's ib and adjusted her pants, she told me, "Grandma says I should say my prayers every day."

I asked her, "Do you think that's a good idea?"

Cody said, "I don't know what prayers is."

I explained, "It's talking to God. It's nice to do any time, especially at bedtime. God likes to hear from you."

Cody was familiar with my father's simple mealtime prayer: "Our Heavenly Father, thank you for this food and all the good things we have. Help us to do right, in Christ's name, amen."

My parents had always modeled love, integrity, and service. They often counseled me to consider how Jesus would handle a problem. Throughout my childhood, new people—even strangers—joined our Sunday dinners and holiday meals, and sometimes people in need moved into our home for a time. But I had little choice about attending Sunday school, weekly church services, Sunday evening youth fellowship meetings, church retreats, Wednesday night church dinners, Bible school, and Christian summer camp. Although I'd prayed all my life, I was cautious about imposing religious practices on Cody. I wanted her to know about God, but I also thought choice was important.

Cody and I decided to say prayers together each night at bedtime.

Tad's sister Becky brought baby Maia for a visit in January and offered her and Robert's home in Bucks Country for our wedding in April. Becky agreed to be matron of honor just as she was my maid of honor when I married her brother.

I told Cody, "I want you to be my flower girl and be right next to me at the wedding. Would you like that?"

She beamed. "Yes, I would."

"You could have a basket of fresh flowers and hand one to each guest."

Cody squealed like she did whenever she was especially excited—a short three-syllable squeal, "oooEEEoow," that I sometimes heard from her room when she was in bed, thinking about something she looked forward to the following day. As the date approached, she awoke each morning with a squeal, saying, "I'm so excited about the wedding!"

Cody came along when I had the blood test required by the Pennsylvania marriage license application. She carried a large pocketbook that "MeeMa" Cornell had given her. I teased Cody, saying that I was a little scared of the blood test.

She said, "Don't worry, Mom. I'm here." Then she added in a consoling tone as I went in for the test, "If you're good, I'll give you something from my purse."

When I returned to the waiting room, Cody said gently, "See? You're okay. It's over now. Do you want someone to talk to?"

I said yes, and she said, "Come here then," motioning me closer.

I sat down in front of Cody and looked at her cherubic smile and twinkling eyes as her arm thrust out. She dropped a tiny wooden Weeble doll in my hand and said, "Talk to this."

We made a quick move to a small duplex and prepared the den for houseguests. When Dennis's mother, Gwen, arrived with her friend Dassie, Cody was thrilled to meet her new grandmother and wanted to stay up late with her the first night. When I finally tucked Cody into bed and finished with prayers, she kept our conversation going, complaining that her bed wasn't comfortable. She wanted a new pillow, one like mine. So I gave her my pillow. She smiled and said that I could have her pillow. With a grin, she added, "But you might want to change the pillowcase. I drooled on it."

She put her head down on her new pillow and sighed, "It's so soft."

As she buried her face deeper, she said it smelled like me. I asked if that was good or bad. Cody said, "It's like perfume." As I kissed her and started to leave, she asked, "What makeup do you wear?"

I said, "Just moisturizer."

"What else?"

"Nothing else."

With a knowing expression, Cody said, "Yes, you do. What about that stuff you put on your armpits?" I smiled and explained why adults use deodorant.

Cody asked, "Can a hairdresser make my hair grow longer?" She wanted to wear her hair in a ponytail, but her hair was too short.

We were back to the difficult "where hair comes from" question. I told Cody it was time to sleep. She sighed. "Okay. Thank you for the pillow."

Cody sat in her wheelchair at my side, holding a basket of daisies as Dennis and I were married outdoors in the sunshine on the creek side of Robert and Becky's home, amidst a circle of relatives and friends. Cody was attentive and ceremonious as Dennis and I recited our vows. After the kiss, she pulled my arm and asked if we were married yet before handing each guest a flower.

After the greetings, music, and toasts, Dennis stood and said to our guests, "On behalf of my wife, daughter, and myself, thank you for sharing today with us."

I saw Cody smile as Dennis called her his "daughter."

Gwen and Dassie stayed with Cody while Dennis and I spent a three-day honeymoon in North Carolina. The kindergarten class gave a recital while we were gone. We were sorry to learn that we'd missed Cody's first public singing performance. Gwen said Cody was terrific.

I hugged Cody as she cried the night Gwen and Dassie left. With tears still wet in her lashes, she began to laugh. "Now I have two dads, three grandmas and grandpas, and even more aunts, uncles, and cousins!"

Chapter 5

Time for a Miracle

"I'm tired, Mommy."

Cody was groggy with a 104.2 degree fever several days after the departure of our houseguests. Her pediatrician said to bring in a urine sample, give Cody cool baths, and alternate aspirin and Tylenol every two hours. The fever went down some. Tad watched her the next day, but at 3:00 p.m., he was unable to wake her. The doctor directed us to the emergency room.

Cody dozed through a battery of tests, a shaved patch of hair, and the draining of a cup of cerebrospinal fluid. Doctors ruled out meningitis, shunt malfunction, pneumonia, and kidney infection. Unable to find another cause for the high fever, the doctor surmised that she had a virus. During Cody's three-day hospital stay, clinicians from the outpatient rehabilitation clinic visited her daily. A physical therapist urged us to rejoin CHOP's coordinated services program. Their new financial assistance service covered leg braces and other medical equipment that might not be reimbursed by health plans. No one asked if Cody was still being seen by a chiropractor, or why we left the CHOP clinic when she was a baby.

The decision to change treatment teams was difficult. Though Cody was covered by insurance that paid many expenses related to her health-care, coverage did not include chiropractics, extra equipment, or many of the supplies and medications she needed. I trusted Dr. Carpenter at Thomas Jefferson University Hospital. However, convinced of the financial advantage and advanced equipment Children's Hospital of Pennsylvania offered, I agreed to transfer Cody's care.

I wrote to Cody's doctors at Jefferson, explaining the decision and thanking them. Dr. Carpenter sent back a kind letter in support of our choice and endorsed the superb care at CHOP. He wrote that his services and advice would always be available to Cody, and that he was genuinely glad to have known our family. Tears filled my eyes reading his last line: "I have admired the way you cared for your child."

Cody crawled into our bedroom one evening and announced, "I want you and Dennis to have a baby. I'd like a big brother."

I smiled. "A baby would be littler than you, sweetie."

"Okay, then I'd like to have a little sister."

I'd already given serious consideration to the advisability of having another child. With Cody's spina bifida and Dennis's brother's hydrocephalus, adoption seemed a safer alternative if we wanted more children. Dennis and I talked briefly about adopting a child, but we decided on a puppy instead. Cody liked the puppy idea but continued to want a sister.

The cockapoo we adopted from the local SPCA had soft hair in shades of gray. Dennis chose her name, Milka, from a novel he was reading. The dogs played together, and Cody pulled the puppy onto her lap. Milka fell asleep with her snout on the arm of the wheelchair as Cody cooed, "Sweet little girl."

Cody received a Master of Rhymes Diploma upon graduation from kindergarten. The school district immediately required her to undergo an evaluation for the appropriateness of starting first grade in the fall. Test results showed that Cody was "within normal age limits" in educational and social development. However, it was suggested that she'd function best in a small structured class to enhance peer interactions. The formal recommendation was for her to attend a "special" school where she could receive physical therapy.

Dennis, Cody, and I visited the special school. Two teachers interviewed Cody. She was talkative that day and the women said they were impressed with her verbal skills. As they further commented upon Cody's intelligence, we learned that most, in addition to being physically disabled, were emotionally disturbed or cognitively impaired.

As Cody transferred into the car and Dennis folded her wheelchair into the trunk, I said, "I don't want Cody in a school where the primary feature she has in common with other students is disability." Dennis agreed. Cody needed to be around all kinds of people, just like in the real world. She needed to go to a public school.

A battle began that entailed many phone calls, letters, and meetings with school officials and administrators. No elementary school in the district had wheelchair ramps or elevator access into or throughout the buildings. A search was on for the school requiring the fewest adaptations to be safe and accessible. Based on the resistance we encountered, I sensed that some folks were not happy with our decision or our persistence. Dennis and I stood firm as options were presented and discussions progressed.

In the course of our correspondence, I found a report in Cody's permanent school record indicating a diagnosis of "brain damage." When questioned, a school official explained that the diagnosis was used to obtain funding of some sort from the state. A school district administrator formally apologized for the inappropriate labeling and promised to change the school record. Such incidents fueled my resolve to keep Cody out of programs that labeled kids "special."

One evening Cody and I lay together in the hammock on our front porch, touching foreheads and cuddling Milka as we chatted about starting first grade. I mentioned something about Tad, and Cody blurted, "Don't talk about him. If you do, by tomorrow morning I'll be very upset, and I'll cry and make you late for work. Don't even *think* about him!"

Tad had moved to Hong Kong that summer to teach English in a Chinese school. He wrote letters to Cody and sent audiotapes. She didn't cry when he first left, but she became upset when she couldn't call him on the phone.

"Okay, we won't talk about Tad. Is there anything else you want to talk about?"

At a clinic visit a few days before, x-rays revealed that Cody's spine was severely curved, "crushing her lungs and displacing her heart." To straighten and fuse her vertebrae at age five would prevent her from growing taller. The alternative was to wear a plastic brace around her torso for several years, removing it only to bathe or change clothes. The plastic mold would be recast as she grew.

Earlier in the day as I spoke on the phone with a friend about the pre-scribed brace, Cody looked up from her toys with a worried expression. I ended the call and asked what was bothering her. She said she was afraid the brace wouldn't fix her spine, and she was mad at me because she had to wear it.

"Me?" I asked in exaggerated surprise.

Cody leaned forward with sudden tears, and anger in her voice. "I should be hitting that *doctor!*"

I empathized. "I bet your doctor will be pretty shocked if we punch him at your next appointment!" Her tears turned to laughter, imagining that.

As we cuddled Milka in the hammock, I asked Cody if she had any other worries about the brace. But she didn't want to talk about the brace, or missing Tad, or anything other than how cute the puppy looked sleeping between us.

Cody sweated only on the left side of her body, no matter how hot the weather. I had to make sure she didn't overheat wearing a T-shirt, the new plastic brace, and a blouse. On very hot days, her left cheek was rosy, flushed, and moist with sweat, while the entire right side of her body was pale and dry. But Cody remained in good spirits through the fittings and the summer heat.

The morning of her sixth birthday, as I adjusted the Velcro straps on her body brace, Cody said in a matter-of-fact voice, "It would be so nice if I could walk. I would get out of bed, put on the robe that MeeMa Gwen brought me, walk downstairs and get myself something to eat and walk back upstairs. That would be nice."

Almost every clinic appointment revealed a new problem or a new feature of an existing problem with Cody's health. I was sick of the ongoing list of complications and poor prognoses for "normalcy" that I heard so often from doctors. I wanted Cody healed. It was apparent that I couldn't depend solely on the medical profession to fix the threats to her well-being. Too much was at stake. I decided it was time to pray for a miracle.

I started reading from the *Children's Bible* to Cody when we said prayers together. The first night I read, I explained to her that Jesus can do anything, even make her walk. Cody immediately said, "Well, tell Jesus to do that!"

"Okay, we will. Starting tonight, we're praying for a miracle so that you get healed."

When it was Cody's turn to pray, she said, "I'm so excited!"

I idly tickled her ankle as she said her prayer. She said, "Hey, Mom, I can feel that."

I interpreted her momentary sensation as a sign that we were on the right track. As a next step, I wrote to my brother Charlie in St. Louis and told him Cody needed a miracle. Charlie believed in miracles; he'd seen many firsthand. He was part of a group that routinely prayed for people who were sick or in some kind of trouble. Charlie called to say that he had a business trip to Philadelphia; he'd see us in a few days.

In the meantime, after meetings, many letters, and a hearing before a judge, we won the battle in time for Cody to start first grade in a "regular" public school. The most accessible elementary school nearby was chosen, and certain adaptations were to be made. An aide was assigned to help Cody with bathroom visits and to make sure she went from place to place during the school day in a timely manner. Architects were to design ramps so Cody could access the gym and recess areas.

When Charlie arrived, we put our hands on Cody and said prayers for her health and healing. As Charlie told stories about healings he'd witnessed, I felt sure that miracles were in the making for Cody.

I prayed for faith and tried not to hope for a miracle for Cody so much as to expect, believe, and be thankful for one. Even though I felt funny admitting to anyone that I expected a miracle, I told a few friends about our prayer request for Cody. I expected to be called a "Jesus freak" and dismissed with rolled eyes, but everyone I told seemed genuinely interested.

I told the osteopath who was treating my chronic neck sprain from the car accident two years before. His face lit up. He said more and more physicians use prayer to heal people, whether the patients knew it or not.

Admittedly, I was not particularly content waiting patiently for God's plan to unfold. I marveled at how patiently Cody dealt with her circumstances. She tolerated so many large and small inconveniences. I watched her strain to reach toys or crayons she dropped. I sensed that, even at age six, she was far wiser than I in some important ways. One day I asked her, "Share your wisdom with me. Teach me how to be patient."

Cody took my question seriously. "I don't know how to be patient, either, Mom. But Dennis must know. Ask him." After a second thought, she added, "When you're feeling impatient and nervous, just ignore it and pretty soon you'll get what you want."

"Cody is a very sweet little girl, but she is not first-grade material," Mrs. R told Dennis and me at the October teacher's conference, "I'm afraid she's feeling frustrated that she can't keep up with others in the class."

I cringed at her description of Cody as "material" and assured Mrs. R that Cody was happy at school. Mrs. R wanted Cody tested at the Child Study Institute to see what experts thought about her school adjustment. That seemed a reasonable idea. By the end of our meeting I could see that Mrs. R had good intentions and wanted what was best for Cody.

That night at bedtime I asked her, "Mrs. R thinks you might not like school. How do you feel about school?"

"I *hate* school! My aide is bossy." She punched her pillow and began to cry, "I miss Tad. Why doesn't he come home?"

I brushed Cody's hair away from her eyes, kissed her and said, "Wait here a minute."

I brought the letter that came that day from Tad and reread it to Cody. He wrote that he wanted her to come to Hong Kong to visit him for a few weeks. She stopped crying, smiled, and said, "He must really miss me."

Dennis and I met with Mrs. R a few weeks later to discuss the Child Study Institute evaluation. The tests indicated that Cody was "a very determined student" who was "age appropriate" with an "average fund of knowledge" and a "sense of humor."

Mrs. R suggested an alternative daily schedule to put less pressure on Cody and ease whatever frustrations she was feeling at school. She began spending the first half of each school day with the first grade class and the second half with the kindergarten class. I took Cody for swimming lessons at the YMCA on Saturday mornings. She said she didn't like swimming much, but she liked the teacher who held onto her in the water. She continued to dislike school; I continued to try to find out why.

At the next clinic appointment, Cody's eyes were examined. The doctor said Cody needed glasses—that she had probably never been able to see the front of the classroom and probably didn't know how to describe what she was missing. Cody was hesitant about wearing glasses, so I asked the doctor to give me a prescription, too. We selected frames together. Cody picked pink ones. We put on our glasses and made faces at each other.

The day Cody wore her glasses to school she told me she saw the blackboard for the first time. Her vision was so improved with glasses, she readily wore them.

The school-hating mystery was further solved when we discovered that Cody was not included in social activities with other kids. Promised ramps had not been built. Cody was left inside with an aide while the rest of the kids played in the gym or outside. Dennis sent a strong letter to the director of pupil services for the school district, reminding him that parts of the school were still inaccessible. [We kept pressing the matter, but the school wasn't entirely accessible until the end of first grade.]

On the way to a friend's house in the car, Cody leaned forward from the backseat and rubbed my neck. I was impressed with the strength of her hands. I said, "Ahh, that feels nice."

She answered, "I've always wanted to do something nice for you, you beautiful woman."

I felt completely adored by Cody. Her high regard for me furthered my commitment to do my best for her. I always thought I fell short. As I studied psychology and human behavior for my job, I read that a point comes in a child's life when complete adoration for the parent is met with the reality of human frailty, and the adored parent comes crashing down from the pedestal. Hoping to offset my inevitable tumble, I told Cody, "I want to have a serious talk with you."

She listened quietly as I looked into her eyes and said, "I love you with my whole heart. I promise to be the best mother I can be, because you are the very best girl in the world. I've made many mistakes, and I'll probably make many more. I'm sincerely sorry for every mistake. And if you're ever mad at me, it's okay, because I will always love you, no matter what. I think God must love me very much to let me have you as my daughter. I love you, babe."

Cody smiled. "I love you, too, Mom. But you're weird."

In December, my brother Charlie called to tell me that seventeen members of his prayer group had prayed together for Cody and felt a confirmation that God held her "in the palm of his hand." He asked if Cody had been baptized.

When Cody was an infant, I thought I might lose her at any time. Remembering a World War II movie on television when I was a kid wherein a soldier baptized his mortally wounded comrade on the battlefield just before he died, I put water on Cody's forehead one evening and baptized her "in the name of the Father, Son, and Holy Spirit." But she had not otherwise been formally baptized.

Cody liked the baptism idea. She planned all of the details for a ceremony. She decided on the music and when to say prayers. She wanted dancing, too. The minister who married Dennis and me met with Cody in early February to discuss the arrangements.

Charlie called from the Philadelphia airport that day during a brief stopover on a business trip. I asked him to tell me more about the prayers for Cody.

He said that when the group prayed in December for Cody's healing, one man experienced a vivid four-part vision: Cody was standing with Jesus beside a stream. Jesus poured a ladle of water over her head and sparkles emanated from it. Then, Cody was strapped in a box underwater in the stream. Finally, Cody and Jesus walked out of the stream together on the other side.

Group members were disturbed by the Cody-in-a-box part. They prayed more, and again felt confirmation of a healing, but no comfort about the third part of the vision. After asking God if there was anything that might be preventing a physical healing, two people had the same vivid vision: Jesus with Cody, Jesus baptizing Cody, Cody breaking straps and getting out of a box in a stream, and Cody and Jesus walking out of the stream on the other side.

The baptism ceremony was the following Saturday at Becky and Robert's house in Bucks County. Becky and Robert became Cody's godparents. The ceremony began with us dancing to a tape recording of "Too Much Heaven" by the Bee Gees. We joined hands in a circle and bowed our heads. Looking at Cody with her eyes shut and her happy smile during a silent prayer, all I could do was thank God for my girl.

Chapter 6

We Are Family

CODY CAME HOME from school one day in March without her winter coat and handed me a note from her teacher asking me to please call her right away. On the phone Mrs. R apologized, saying, "I have no idea what happened to it. I feel terrible about it. I'm so sorry." Then she laughed, repeating Cody's response to her concern about the missing coat: "Don't worry, Mrs. R. It's okay. I'm a rich kid."

I laughed, too. Cody was hardly a rich kid, but I felt terrific knowing she felt like one.

Dennis's father had a fatal heart attack that winter. Dennis couldn't go to Australia for the funeral, so he sent money for his mother to visit us again. Gwen arrived in April and brought Dennis's younger brother, Mark.

Cody had heard about Mark for years. She'd seen the Australian newspaper articles about the famous boy—the first in the world to survive with a shunt in his brain.

Mark, now twenty, was tall and shy, with a simple manner and particular tastes. He was especially sensitive to sound, most likely a side effect of the hydrocephalus he was diagnosed with at birth. His head was larger than average, but at six-feet-six, everything about Mark was large. From the moment he smiled and leaned down to say hello to Cody, she loved her uncle. She sang, "*I love you Mar-kie, oh yes, I do. I don't love anyone as much as you.*"

One evening as Gwen, Dennis, Cody, and I sat talking in the living room, Cody's eyes widened in fear seeing Mark stumble as he came down the staircase. His eyes rolled up and his body shuddered. Cody remained brave and still as Dennis ran up the steps and braced his body in front of Mark to keep him from falling as he convulsed in a seizure.

I rushed to call our doctor, who said to take Mark to nearby Philadelphia Osteopathic Hospital. Dennis spoke softly and helped Mark to our car. Gwen went along and I stayed home with Cody. I remained outwardly unruffled so as not to scare her further, but my stomach churned.

She asked, "Is it okay to cry now?"

I said yes, and Cody burst into despairing sobs. She cried and cried for her uncle. We cuddled in bed with the dogs and said prayers. Cody refused to sleep until Dennis called after 2:00 a.m. to say Mark would be okay. Cody cheered, "Yay! Thank you, God!"

Mark had brain surgery the following morning to implant a new shunt, and was hospitalized for eight days. After his release, Cody patted Mark's arm and said, "I know how you feel. My shunt broke down, too, one time."

When Gwen and Mark returned to Australia, his physician apologetically admitted that Mark would not have survived if his emergency had occurred in Australia at that time. I felt angel shivers, realizing what a miracle it was that twenty years after the implant of his first, newsworthy shunt, the surgery that saved his life was in America with us.

Cody performed the role of a tree in the first grade play. She said her lines in a loud voice, needing only a couple of prompts. After the play, Mrs. R told Dennis and me about a budding romance "everyone" in first grade was talking about between Cody and a boy in her class. She and Peter exchanged love notes and drew pictures for each other. Mrs. R invited us to help chaperone an overnight camping trip with the entire class during the last week of school. There we saw firsthand how Peter treated Cody.

The first-graders were an energetic group. I never had to worry about Cody getting into the kind of trouble kids do who walk, run, and climb, but these kids were not still even for a moment. Dennis and I plucked them out of trees and applied bandages to cuts and scrapes. But Peter stayed near Cody with one hand resting on the handle of her wheelchair. He held her marshmallow over the campfire, and she glowed in his attention.

By the time everyone was tucked into sleeping bags, Dennis and I were ready to drop. We were in a tent with Mrs. R and her husband when we heard, "Mrs. R! Matthew threw up!" The camp came alive again as kids ran from tents and yelled *Eewwwww!*

I noticed the next day that Cody allowed Peter to push her wheelchair. He rushed to pick up anything she dropped. Mrs. R took Peter aside and told him it was important for him to treat Cody like other children and not do so much for her. As sweet as his helpful intentions were, it was a bad idea for Cody to develop an expectation that others would do things for her.

We often found it necessary to explain to friends and relatives that it was more helpful and respectful to let Cody do for herself the things she could do on her own. That would make her strong, confident, and better able to care for herself. This was a lesson retaught many times to everyone in Cody's life. Though the concept was difficult for a child to grasp, Peter was careful after that to help Cody only when asked.

Our summer was busy. Cody attended day camp. Dennis worked on his Ph.D. dissertation and taught part-time. I worked full time and spent non-work time with Cody's exercise regimen, body-brace equipment, skincare, bowel and bladder health, and drives to New Jersey for her chiropractor appointments.

A clinician suggested sending Cody to a residential facility for a month to learn bowel and bladder program skills. I'd taken similar advice the summer Cody was five. She'd been referred to a seashore camp for four weeks to slim down and develop body strength to increase her mobility. She was miserably homesick the first ten days and gained weight. I felt guilty for that decision and wouldn't repeat my mistake.

I continued to research homeopathic remedies and nutritional supplements. A naturopath recommended rubbing warm peanut oil on Cody's back each evening, to stimulate her nerves, I think. Cody and I talked while I massaged her. She was lonely for other children. She called the little girl across the street every day to invite her to play. Melanie came for a few minutes twice, when none of her other friends were around, and only then, she told us, because her father "forced" her. Cody's feelings were hurt. She and I said a prayer for her to find more friends.

A few weeks before Cody turned seven, I began to experience a light-headed, queasy fear, usually at night—a restless sense that all was not right with the world. My boss, a gifted psychotherapist and dear friend, suggested that I might be experiencing anxiety attacks from taking on too much responsibility. I didn't see what I could do about that.

Our family made a quick half-mile move to a more cheerful and spacious house across the street from good friends with three sons who Cody adored. Two were old enough to babysit her after school. The move was temporary in that we planned to relocate within a year to wherever Dennis's first "real" academic job took us.

My panic attacks continued, but Cody's joy and faith were contagious. While planning her birthday party in August, I heard her tell a friend on the phone about our prayers for a healing miracle. "Wouldn't it be great if I could walk on my birthday? One leg would move, then the other. Can you just imagine everyone's faces? And me saying, 'Mother, Father, everyone! I have a surprise for you!'"

Tad returned to Philadelphia for an extended visit in time for Cody's party. He brought her gifts from Hong Kong and took her to the theater.

Cody awoke on her birthday and announced, "When I was four, I wanted to be five. When I was five, I wanted to be six. When I was six, it was perfect. And now I'm seven!"

That night, Cody and I prayed as usual for faith in more miracles not yet seen. After I read a passage in her *Children's Bible*, she became serious and said, "I hope I can talk to you about this . . . I *am* seven."

"What is it, honey?" I expected a Bible story question.

"About that stuff you do under the covers with Dennis . . ." She paused and asked, "Why do you keep doing it?"

There was only one instance I knew of when Cody had any idea that

Dennis and I did anything under the covers other than sleep. She was five at the time, and we'd not heard her push open the bedroom door. We were startled to see her on the floor propped on her elbows, watching us intently with her chin resting on her hands. Before Dennis or I could respond, Cody had grinned and said, "Do that again!" We all laughed. She didn't ask anything further at the time, so we left it at that. Now she wanted details.

Cody listened carefully as I explained how and why people have sex; then she said firmly, "I would never, *ever* do that."

I reminded her of some foods, such as olives, that she once hated and now loved. She agreed that it was possible for her to change her mind about some things, but not *that*.

"By the time you grow up and are ready to do it, you'll like it. Besides, sweetie, if you ever want to have a baby, you'll have to do it at least once."

Cody frowned in thought. "Well, I guess I'll have to do it once."

Less than a month after her birthday, Cody yelled, "Mom! I can move my foot!"

She wiggled her left foot again and again to show me; then she wiggled it for Dennis when he came home from work. "I knew I'd have a miracle! I think my left leg is healing. I bet someday I'll walk with only a crutch."

Prior to that, Cody had not been able to move either leg or foot. She'd felt my tickle on a few occasions, but never a consistent response. The only movement in her lower extremities was an occasional involuntary leg spasm that could throw her backward if she was sitting on the floor. Muscles in her left leg twitched if her leg was touched by something cold, and she sometimes described unusual sensations.

I asked her, "What does it feel like to wiggle your foot?"

"It feels like moving furniture into a new house."

Over the next few days, Cody described feelings in her legs above the knee. I tested her reactions with her eyes covered and asked her when she could feel my touch. Her responses were accurate. Dennis and Cody and I had moments of excitement and moments of calm wonder. Friends and relatives had mixed reactions. Some were shocked, amazed, or impressed. A few were mildly interested, unsure what to make of it. A friend at work advised me to keep a written record. We didn't mention anything to Cody's doctors about the new movement in her foot. The small change didn't affect her overall abilities. But it was a change.

Cody's faith in ultimate victory over her health issues influenced everyone around her. Dennis had not attended church since his youth, but now he invited Cody to join him and they went each Sunday to St. Matthias Church two blocks away.

Though I was raised Presbyterian, I was attracted to the rituals, incense, and beauty of the Catholic Church. Now that Cody was attending church with Dennis, I decided to meet with a priest at Saint Matthias to learn how to become Catholic.

The elderly priest leaned forward and spoke in a firm voice, "First, my dear, you need to understand that the day you *die* will be the best day of your life!"

I didn't recall much he said after that. But after his one-hour monologue, I decided it wasn't the right time to become Catholic.

Pope John Paul visited Philadelphia in early October and Tad heard him speak at St. Charles Seminary. Within days, Tad confided that he felt he might have a spiritual calling to become a monk or a priest. Even though we weren't married in a Catholic church, our marriage had to be officially "annulled" in order for him to pursue the priesthood. He took care of the annulment process, but he still had "parental obligations." When Dennis expressed interest in legally adopting Cody, the way was paved for Tad to pursue his potential spiritual calling. I had trusted that Tad would care for Cody if I died, and I also trusted Dennis. But I held a private belief that I would not die as long as Cody needed me. More and more, I thought that to care for, defend, and love her was my purpose in life. Dennis and I met with a lawyer to initiate adoption proceedings.

Cody and I took Dennis out for dinner for his birthday in mid-November. The plastic brace under Cody's smock kept her posture straight as she leaned forward and ate like a grownup. She held her fork with her fingers fanned out as though holding a delicate teacup.

Over her shoulder, I saw Jim O'Brien, a local TV weatherman, dining with another man in a far corner of the restaurant. Throughout the meal Cody whispered, "Is he still here?" When we finished eating, I showed Cody where to look, so that she could see Jim O'Brien as we wheeled from the restaurant. At the exit, Cody stopped, turned her wheelchair around and said, "Come with me, Mom. I want to ask Jim O'Brien if we're going to have snow flurries tonight."

I said, "I don't think so. No, thank you." I hoped she'd abandon the idea, but Cody wheeled back into the restaurant and maneuvered through the maze of tables. With strong arms, she was fairly adept at guiding her chair without banging into things. I slumped onto a barstool near the entrance while Dennis retrieved our coats. A bartender asked for my order.

"Nothing, thanks. My daughter is asking Jim O'Brien about snow flurries."

The bartender smiled, but a hostess standing with her hand on her hip commented, "He hates being bothered." (I hoped he wouldn't yell at a seven-year-old in a wheelchair.)

I heard laughing from the restaurant. A waitress came out and said, "That was cute."

Cody wheeled toward me, grinning. "Jim O'Brien wants to meet you, Mom!"

"You're kidding, right?"

She paused before answering, "Yeah, I'm kidding."

I gave Cody a mock scowl and said, "You little creep, you," and the bartender laughed.

Cody giggled as Dennis helped her on with her coat. In the parking lot, I asked her to tell me about her conversation with Jim O'Brien.

"I just wheeled up to him and he said, 'Who are you?' and I said 'Cody.' I looked at the other man and Jim O'Brien said, 'He's just my boss.' And the boss asked me if I have a boss."

Cody had answered, "Yeah, two. My mom and dad . . . do you want to meet my mom?" She apparently asked this several times before Jim O'Brian finally said yes.

"Okay, I'll go get her." Cody had spun around and wheeled away.

As I steered the car toward the parking lot exit, I turned to look at Cody. "Do you mean Jim O'Brien *is* waiting to meet me?"

"Yes." She looked up with innocent eyes. At that moment, Jim O'Brien and his boss walked out of the restaurant. As I steered past the entrance, Cody rolled down the car window and shouted, "Goodbye, Jim! My mother was too scared to meet you!"

She giggled off and on the whole way home.

During Thanksgiving vacation, Cody and Dennis were wrestling on the living room floor when we heard a loud crack as she rolled sideways. The roughhousing stopped instantly. We looked carefully at both legs for signs of injury. As I bent Cody's left leg, Dennis and I cringed as we heard grinding. Her leg was broken above the knee. She hadn't felt it break, and she said it didn't hurt. We spent the next six hours in an emergency room.

The lack of pain on Cody's part allowed us each to remain in good spirits despite waiting, interviews, x-rays, and the application of a plaster cast she had to wear for eight weeks. Dennis was mortified to have caused her broken leg. Cody took delight in teasing him and telling the medical folks, "My dad broke my leg." She laughed every time she said it, as nurses looked us up and down. That made us all laugh. We were giddy with silliness.

Being in an emergency room was so much easier when it wasn't a matter of life and death, and no one was in pain. When we were ready to go home, Dennis extended the foot pedal on the wheelchair to support Cody's leg. Her foot peeked out of the bottom of the cast. She pointed and smiled. "Look, I can still wiggle my foot!"

Cody's love life had new complications in second grade. She had not seen Peter over the summer and rarely mentioned him that fall. I wondered if their affection had faded. She talked about a new boy, Ryan, who gave her jewelry, stuffed toys, and love notes.

On Parents' Day, Dennis and I met Ryan. He was a handsome, athletic eight-year-old, a real macho ladies' man, I thought. Mrs. R was Cody's teacher again in second grade. She told us she had a conversation with Ryan about the importance of not doing so much for Cody—the same talk as the previous year with Peter.

Ryan and Cody spent hours on the phone. She was invited to his house and he came to our house. He invited her to the ice-skating rink and baseball games. His presents continued. My parents visited at Christmas and, observing Ryan, Dad said he'd never seen a child so solicitous.

Cody coughed and Ryan ran to get her a drink of water. I followed Ryan to the kitchen and said, "You know, you don't need to do so much for Cody. She has to be very good at pushing her wheelchair and reaching for things. She won't always have you around when she drops something or needs a drink."

Ryan said he understood. He told me, "I pray for Cody every day."

Soon I found out that Peter was still, or perhaps back, in the picture. I heard snippets of phone conversation and occasional comments from Cody. Peter invited her to his house, but she came home early. Without knowing details, I wondered if Cody's behavior towards Peter was affected by how accustomed she'd become to Ryan's doting. So I asked her what was going on. She said both boys were jealous; they argued. She blurted, "I'm torn between two lovers!"

She thought Peter was the most jealous. To make him feel better, she'd told him she liked him best. I explained to Cody, "It's okay to like both boys. You don't have to pick a favorite. It's good to have lots of friends."

A few days later I learned more when Peter came to our house after school. I arrived home from work to find Cody teary and Peter flustered. Dennis was busy in the study and hadn't noticed a problem. Peter asked to "speak privately" with me. He told me what was going on, and his face flushed in anger as he said, "I hate it when Cody orders me around like a slave."

I told Peter, "I think Cody needs to hear how you feel."

When Peter told Cody exactly what he'd said to me, she responded sincerely, "I'm sorry, Peter. I won't boss you around anymore."

With that, Peter and Cody were okay again and resumed their play. But after dinner I heard Cody tell Peter, "I love you, and that Ryan is a brat."

I said, "It's not nice to tell Peter that you hate Ryan, especially since it isn't true. Ryan is a good friend, and so is Peter. I'm sure he doesn't mind knowing you have more than one friend."

Peter nodded in agreement.

Cody admitted, "I like both Peter and Ryan."

Peter scowled and said, "The Ryan subject should just be avoided!"

When Cody scooted into bed that night, she said she felt much better after telling Peter the truth. We discussed what it's like to have two friends who don't like each other much, and how maybe for now it's better not to talk so much about one in front of the other.

I recalled the summer before when Cody was so lonely. We'd prayed for her to find more friends. I now thanked God that Cody had friend-ships with Peter and Ryan. Stephanie, the other classmate in a wheelchair, had recently called Cody; and Matthew, the one who threw up in the tent, had asked to come over to play.

Cody lost a friend from school that winter. Mahjong died a few days after Christmas. I didn't know what kind of cancer she had, but her medica-tions changed Mahjong from slender and delicate to chubby and round. This was the first death of a person Cody knew; she was very sad. We had a few conversations about diseases and death.

Mrs. R said that she and the other teachers sometimes referred to Cody as "Sarah Bernhardt" because she tended to be "emotional and dramatic." She also had some typical Virgo qualities according to astrology books I'd read, such as an exaggerated concern about germs and health issues. Cody had many genuine medical problems, so I took her concerns seriously, no matter how dramatically described, and tried not to react to her fear with fears of my own. When Cody was sick, I calmly asked her questions. I explained things to her simply and without drama. We talked together until we figured out the problem.

One winter evening at bedtime, Cody said, "I want to talk to you. It's serious, Mom." Her eyebrows pressed together and her voice shook. "I didn't want to have to tell you this . . . I think I have cancer."

I asked, "Why do you think you have cancer?"

Cody's broken leg had healed and her cast was gone. She looked up at me with a face ready to crumple into tears, and pointed to a small freckle on her knee.

"Cody, that's a freckle, a very normal-looking freckle." I unbuttoned my shirt and said, "Look at my chest, my arms, my back. I have lots of freckles. It's normal for you to have freckles. I'm surprised you don't have more freckles, considering you're my little girl!"

Her face smoothed in relief.

During a visit from Ryan, he and Cody had so sweet an exchange; I wished I could have stood and stared or taken a picture. I walked back and forth, straightening the kitchen as though I hardly noticed, so as not to disturb their tender interaction.

Ryan had his knees between Cody's feet on her wheelchair footrests as he leaned forward in a hug. Cody's arms were around him, and her fingers were laced together behind his neck. Her eyes were shut and her face tilted against his cheek. Ryan idly rocked her wheels back and forth with his hands while they chattered to each other and to me.

Cody's formal adoption required an appearance in court in February. The night before, she awoke crying. Dennis and I both went to see what was wrong. She'd had a bad dream and she was thirsty. I brought her a cup of water. She took a sip, smiled at Dennis, and said, "Pretty soon you'll be my real dad!"

He hugged Cody and we all kissed goodnight again. I dreamt that Cody could walk. In the dream, I held her right hand as she took her first steps, and I thanked God.

In the morning, Cody, Tad, Dennis, and I drove together to Montgomery County Courthouse. We sat in a dimly lit courtroom with high ceilings and dark, wood-paneled walls, rails, and benches. Flags with gold rope tassels perched on either side of the judge's raised bench. Somber and churchlike, we spoke in whispers as we waited for the robed judge to speak. We were told when to stand and sit. The judge asked a few simple questions of each of us to make sure we all agreed to the adoption. The entire proceeding took less than fifteen minutes.

We left the courthouse, cheering and singing, "We Are Family," as we held hands in a line and pulled Cody's wheelchair across the parking lot. Cody sang her own words, "*We are fa-mi-ly, Mommy, Dennis, Tad-die and me.*"

Chapter 7

Oz to Minnesota

DENNIS ACCEPTED AN OFFER to teach in the business school at the University of Minnesota starting that fall. When I asked the physicians at CHOP about the transfer of Cody's medical care to the Minneapolis/St. Paul area, they suggested clinicians at the University of Minnesota Hospital. Tad stayed with Cody in June while Dennis and I flew to the Twin Cities to find a place to live.

We found a house to rent in South Minneapolis with a wood-burning stove, two upstairs bedrooms, and an upper back porch. Cody was not an overweight seven-year-old, but I couldn't lift her up stairs without hurting myself. My neck sprain wasn't fully healed from the car accident; I still had frequent headaches and pain. Dennis said not to worry; he'd carry Cody up the stairs until we could find a place on one level.

I turned in my resignation at work, sad to leave a job I loved and colleagues who were also close friends. Cody was in a similar situation. Ryan's family hosted a goodbye party and invited the entire class, the principal, and Mrs. R. Each child presented Cody with a homemade card with messages about how much she would be missed, and signed with hearts, X's, and O's.

Dennis arranged for us to go to Australia for a few weeks during the summer before our move to Minnesota. Cody was eager to meet the rest of her Australian relatives and see her grandmother and Uncle Mark again.

Before the trip, Cody's urologist showed me how to use a Foley catheter so Cody wouldn't need to leave her airplane seat during flights. The catheter could stay in place, draining urine into a bag that I could empty as needed. There was one for the long trip to Australia and one for each separate flight on the return trip. We planned a stop in Los Angeles to take Cody to Disneyland. Our journey to "Oz" (as Dennis called Australia) had one plane change and stops in San Francisco, Hawaii, and the Fiji Islands before finally landing in Sydney.

Cody had flown on airplanes before, but not over an ocean or for such a long distance. She brought reading material, coloring books, her music tape player and headset. Dennis used an airplane aisle chair to wheel Cody to our row on the plane. She slid sideways to her seat, and the wheelchair was stowed in the baggage compartment.

The airplane leaving San Francisco was large, with two aisles. We sat in a center section with five seats across. The older lady next to us didn't seem to mind Cody's ongoing chatter. That was a blessing because we were packed in tight. I hoped Cody would nod off the same way she did on long car rides.

I underestimated the excitement that kept her talking nonstop until just before the plane landed on each portion of the trip: "I can't wait to see MeeMa Gwen. I'll get to play with Uncle Mark. I drew him a picture. I'll get to ride the bus with him. I saw a kangaroo before. I wish Ryan came with us. I miss Sadie and Milka. How big is MeeMa Gwen's dog? I'm excited to see my cousins. Do they have a dog? Hey, Mom, are you asleep?"

The plane traveled over the South Pacific in continuous daylight as we followed the morning sun halfway around the world. Before landing in Fiji we were served a breakfast of fresh fruit with flowers and a glass of guava juice. Flight attendants came down the aisles with trays of steamy rolled towels. With tongs, each passenger was given a hot towel to freshen hands and face.

I emptied Cody's urine bag once or twice on each segment of the trip by covering both of our laps with a blanket, draining the urine into a soft-drink can that I emptied in the airplane bathroom. The bag remained strapped to Cody's leg under her long cotton pants and wasn't otherwise visible.

Without access to Cody's wheelchair until landing in Sydney, leaving the confined space and the stale air in the plane between each four-hour portion of the trip meant using the aircraft stairs that were wheeled to the airplane doors. Dennis carried Cody up and down the steps and then I carried her as long as I could. Cody clutched onto me tightly to make it easier for me to carry her as we entered the duty-free shop in Fiji.

While turning around in the narrow aisle, I bumped into the back of an Australian man who swung around and looked like he was about to lunge at me when he stopped and, in the broadest Australian accent I'd ever heard, said, "Oye thawt yoo was moy woyf and oye was abeowt to wek 'er bek!" (I thought you was my wife, and I was about to whack her back!)

I smiled and apologized. Cody giggled as we left the store to find Dennis, who was off taking pictures. Fiji smelled like fresh flowers. We took deep breaths of fragrant air and stood in the sunshine before boarding the plane for the final flight to Oz.

Cody fell sound asleep just as the plane landed in Sydney.

Traveling with Cody, we were the first to board airplanes. She enjoyed that advantage. Conversely, we were the last to exit the plane after Cody's wheelchair was brought up from the baggage compartment. Once deplaned and through customs, we were met by Dennis's teenage sister, Leanne, who drove us south to Fairy Meadow, where she and Mark lived with their mother. Though winter in Australia, the temperature was sixty-eight degrees. The sky was clear and blue. I pointed out to Cody that we were driving on the left side of the road.

Gwen insisted that Dennis and I use her bedroom during our visit. Cody slept on a veranda next to a window of our room so we could chat at night. On her bed was a beautiful quilt Gwen made for Cody. Gwen showed us prize-winning cross-stitched pieces she'd made since her husband died. She spent part of each day teaching Cody how to cross-stitch.

Until the third week in July, we visited family and friends and took day trips up and down the coast to sightsee and watch for kangaroos. A stiff wind was blowing the day we took a train into Sydney. Our compartment had four seats on each side. I sat across from Dennis and Cody. The other seats were occupied. No one spoke during the ride except Cody. As the other passengers read books or newspapers, she directed her chatter to no one in particular.

"I like this train. See Dad, I'm riding backwards. I think my cousin Richard is handsome, and Melissa is so cute. I want to see all my cousins again tomorrow." She stopped to look out the window and said, "I wonder what Tad is doing. I'm lucky to have two dads. I am the only kid I know with two dads."

At that, the other passengers looked up at Dennis, Cody, and me. Noticing their attention, Cody said, "Hello." Without speaking, they each went back to their reading.

Our time in Australia was almost at an end by the time we visited Raywinkle's, an animal preserve where Cody saw mobs of kangaroos speckling the hillsides. She held crunchy food nuggets in her outstretched hand and a medium-sized kangaroo nibbled the snack.

A man from the preserve brought a baby koala to show Cody. The wooly marsupial looked like a stuffed toy bear with eyes like black marbles. His long sharp claws clung to the man's thick elbow-length leather gloves. He told us that the koala is a gentle creature, but his claws looked so menacing that Cody didn't want to touch him.

Adjusting to the fifteen-hour time change had taken two weeks, so Dennis and I decided to break up the return trip to ease jetlag on the way home. After our taste of Fiji at the airport, we thought it would be nice to visit a tropical island. Dennis arranged a three-day stop in American Samoa and an extra day in California.

Rain poured all three days we were in Samoa on the outskirts of Pago Pago. We spent the entire time on the open-sided terraces of the aptly named Rainmaker Hotel. Dennis and I read and Cody colored or worked on her cross-stitch project.

In sunny, dry Los Angeles, we found a motel in Anaheim and spent the day at Disneyland. Bathroom facilities were excellent and almost everything in the park was wheelchair accessible. Cody was invited to the front of every line. The day was wonderful except for a seemingly endless ride in small boats through an exhibit originally created for the 1964 New York World's Fair. A few hundred dolls dressed as people from different countries danced and sang, "*It's a small world after all.*"

Cody cried, "Get me out of here," and buried her face in my shirt.

Exhausted by dinnertime, we decided to go back to the motel. We picked up sandwiches and fruit at a grocery store on the way. The night was swelteringly hot and the room's air conditioner didn't work. Cody sat on one bed, wearing only an incontinent brief and her back brace (over a T-shirt). Dennis and I finally took all our clothes off and sat on the other bed, watching television and fanning the air with wet washcloths.

Before going to sleep I gathered wrappers from dinner and peeked out our motel room door, which faced the parking lot. The garbage can sat about eight feet from our door. I wrapped myself in a towel and stepped out quickly to discard our trash. As I turned, a couple appeared, screaming at each other in French. The woman slapped the man's face, ran past me into *our* room, and slammed the door. The man stormed off in the other direction.

Left standing outside in a towel, I was not sure what to do. Clutching my towel, I walked across to the motel lobby and told the man at the registration desk what happened. He called our room and asked, "Sir, is there a strange woman in your room?"

Dennis answered, "Yes, there is."

The motel man asked, "What's going on?"

"I don't know." Then a pause. "Ah, she left."

I thanked the motel man and returned to the room. Dennis and Cody told me what occurred in my absence: When the woman had entered the room, she sobbed and peeked out the window curtain. Dennis and Cody had remained still. Dennis slowly reached for something to cover himself, but the only thing close by was a damp washcloth.

Apparently the woman didn't pay much attention to Dennis or Cody. She ran out the door as suddenly as she came. Cody giggled so continuously, telling me how Dennis looked trying to cover his privates with a washcloth, that it took her several minutes to finish the story. She couldn't decide which predicament was funnier: Dennis trying to cover himself with a washcloth, or me stuck outside with only a towel.

Sandwiched in the weeks between our return home and our departure for Minnesota, Cody's shunt broke down. It was hardly more than three years since her Valentine's Day shunt revision. Although the emergency aspect of this hospital experience was frightening, the incision behind Cody's right ear was not large and did not require much hair to be shaved. I wondered if our recent air travel was a factor, but the neurosurgeon didn't think so. Cody thought it "convenient" for the shunt breakdown to occur while we still lived near Children's Hospital rather than during our trip.

Cody wanted to celebrate her eighth birthday before our move to Minnesota. Her idea was to have an art show. After attending a painting exhibit of mine the previous spring she announced that she wanted to be an artist. We taped a dozen of her finest works to railings on our front porch along with streamers and balloons. She sold her paintings and drawings for a dime or a quarter to relatives at the party.

Tad saw us off the final morning. Our car was packed with houseplants, a television, and enough clothes and supplies for four days. The wheelchair was folded in the trunk, and Milka and Sadie sat on pillows in the backseat with Cody for the 1,200-mile drive northwest.

We arrived in Minneapolis one day before the moving truck, plugged in the TV, and slept that night on the bedroom carpet. The next week was spent arranging for Cody to start third grade in a "regular" elementary school. Our experience in Pennsylvania had prepared us to expect a struggle, but the nearest elementary school in South Minneapolis had a third grade classroom on the main level, so the process was easier than expected. Cody was the first child in a wheelchair to attend Seward School.

My next project was to make our home more accessible. Both entries to our house were up a few steps. I made calls and learned about an organization in St. Paul that helped families with children who were disabled. For a reduced fee, a carpenter built a ramp from the sidewalk to our kitchen door.

Cody missed school on a day in early October to attend her first appointment at the University of Minnesota Hospital Myelodysplasia

Clinic. During the lengthy evaluation, a physician told us that Cody's joints were contracting; she couldn't fully straighten her legs. She hadn't worn leg braces in a year. She needed another hip-and-knee-release surgery to improve her positioning, after which she could try a new standing frame.

Cody told the physician, "No!"

The doctor didn't press the point, but he stressed that wearing leg braces was important.

As I put Cody to bed that night, I sat next to her and tucked the covers around her shoulders. We'd just hung a new poster of Mork from Ork above her bed, and her new guinea pig, Dassie Jane, was scratching around in the cedar chips in a large glass fish tank.

Cody said with conviction, "Those doctors have a nerve! When somebody says no, they should take no for an answer. They're not as smart as God!"

"Don't worry about it," I said. "We'll get more information before deciding what to do. The surgery might be a very good idea, and it might not. Can I hear your song?"

Cody had been listening to the theatrical soundtrack of *Annie* ever since Tad took her to the musical in Philadelphia. She sang, "*The sun'll come out to-mor-row . . .*"

After she sang all the verses, I said, "That was beautiful! You know all the words!"

Cody beamed. "Michaela, a second grade teacher, thinks I'm very good, and she said she's heard a lot of little kids sing."

"Well, I agree. You are good."

Cody looked at the dogs and started to laugh. Sadie and Milka sat side by side in front of Dassie Jane's glass tank as if they were watching television.

Cody wrote to Ryan, inviting him for a visit. His parents were willing to let him fly to Minneapolis for the Thanksgiving holiday if we'd take him to a Catholic church on Sunday.

My new painting teacher had invited us to his home for Thanksgiving dinner. George was a Native American who walked with a limp. He was a man of few words, but whenever George saw Cody he engaged her in conversation. He told her he'd been bedridden as a boy for a year with his legs in casts due to a problem with his hips. George and his wife Hazel, also an accomplished artist, welcomed us warmly on Thanksgiving Day.

Before dinner, George held a long peace pipe with tobacco from his brother's reservation land up north. George lifted the lit pipe in each direction and handed it around the table. He told us the smoke would carry our prayers heavenward to the Great Spirit. Cody and Ryan in turn carefully sipped a little smoke from the pipe and passed it on. Before wrapping the pipe in colorful cloth, George wrote each guest's name in his record of those who'd smoked with him.

Our hosts, the food, the stunning artwork, and the pipe ceremony made this Thanksgiving outstanding. At bedtime, after the Lord's Prayer, and a Hail Mary for our Catholic guest, each of us added a personal prayer. Ryan prayed for a miracle healing for Cody.

At nearby St. Albert's Church on Sunday morning, Cody wanted to take communion with Ryan. But I'd heard that the Catholic Church didn't condone taking communion there if you weren't Catholic. After Ryan flew home, Cody again mentioned wanting communion. So I suggested we go to the rectory after school the next day to ask a priest about it.

A friendly man named Father Dan met with Cody and me. He invited us into a room near the main hall of the rectory and we sat together.

I began, "My daughter would like to take communion."

Father Dan smiled and said, "We can arrange that." He turned to Cody and said, "First, I need to ask you one important question, Cody. Do you know the difference between ordinary bread and communion bread?"

Cody replied, "Yes."

"Then you may have your first communion this Sunday."

Father Dan turned to me and asked, "Are you Catholic?"

"I've thought about becoming Catholic. I talked to a priest in Philadelphia. It sounded complicated and involved a lot of formal instruction."

Father Dan said, "Well, I see no reason to make it a difficult process. If you want to be Catholic, you can join with Cody on Sunday."

Surprised, I asked, "How is that possible? I don't know everything it means to be a Catholic."

With a warm smile he said, "You may not know everything about being a Catholic, but you'll be no less a Catholic."

Cody and I each had our first communion at St. Albert's that Sunday. The "affirmation of faith" was easy to agree to; it was basic Christianity as I knew it. But at the end, the priest asked if I agreed with all the teachings of the Catholic Church. I wasn't expecting that question. I said "yes" out loud, but privately assured God that I wasn't certain about that part.

The church was full of friendly folks. Several people hugged Cody and me after the service. From then on, Dennis, Cody, and I attended church at St. Albert's each week and sat in the second row near the side entrance.

Chapter 8

That's Incredible

As DENNIS PACKED in January for a week in Massachusetts to work on a project with his research partner, television programming was interrupted to announce that the Iran hostage crisis ended after 444 days. On our way to the airport I explained to Cody why this news was a cause for celebration. We went to the gate with Dennis and waved goodbye as he boarded the plane.

Back at home Cody spoke soothingly to Milka, "Now, don't miss Dennis. He'll be home soon. And Tad's coming tomorrow."

I asked Cody how she wanted to spend our evening. Quoting a TV commercial, she said, "Mom, let's celebrate the moments of our lives and have a cup of tea." So we did.

Tad's arrival in Minneapolis was perfectly timed. With Dennis away, I needed his help to carry Cody upstairs. Tad had joined a Trappist monastery in upstate New York. Abbey rules were strict regarding visitors—family members only, and visits were limited to three days per year. Tad wanted to visit Cody before moving to the cloistered community.

Cody and I waited at the gate and watched airplanes land. Tad's morning flight was late. Several folks waited near us, looking out the big windows. Cody spoke in a voice loud enough for those around us to hear, "Isn't this great, Mom? One dad leaves on a plane yesterday, and another dad comes today!"

All faces turned in our direction. I looked at Cody and crossed my eyes.

She burst out laughing even though she wasn't sure why her comment attracted attention.

While Dennis was away, Cody and I experienced a taste of what our original family might have been like had we'd stayed together. Tad knew how to make Cody dissolve in laughter. He'd perfected a skill he used in a high school play wherein his character said a line before falling flat on his face. He went into Cody's closet and shut the door. As the door slowly opened, Tad's stiffened body fell forward, landing facedown on the floor. She begged him to fall out of the closet again and again. She laughed just as hard every time. Sometimes Cody threw a pillow at him as he fell. He screamed in mock alarm, and she laughed harder.

To get Tad close enough for a surprise tickle or kiss, Cody feigned indifference and said, "Hey, Tad, come here a minute." She wiggled a finger for him to come near her. He moved closer and closer until she could reach out to tickle his stomach. He let out a little scream and sprang backwards. Tad fell for her ruse whenever she tried it.

At bedtime each night, we sang "Circle Game," Cody's favorite of the songs we'd sung to her each night in the big house. At the end of Tad's stay, Cody asked when she'd see him again. He promised to request permission for a Christmas visit.

Dennis came home stressed from his trip. His research project had received media coverage, and he was nervous about the attention and expectations it suggested. As an assistant professor in the business school, teaching was only one-third of his job. The more time-consuming aspect of his work was the research that resulted in published articles in academic journals. His new work schedule included evenings, weekends, and additional travel in the coming months to Quebec, San Francisco, and Washington. This was just the beginning. Dennis's new research projects entailed more and more travel.

At a spring clinic appointment, the tendons in Cody's legs were tighter. The doctor wanted to schedule the hip-and-knee release operation for the summer because she'd be in the hospital for three weeks and spend four more weeks lying down. The operation could be done at Gillette

Children's Hospital in St. Paul, a hospital that specialized in treating kids with disabilities. But before an appointment could be made, Cody's shunt broke down. She spent two days in the University Hospital. Another brain surgery after only a year was alarming, but Cody recovered and was back home so quickly that it was more like a bad dream.

On Cody's first monthly visit to Gillette, we saw that the outpatient clinic was designed for complete accessibility and patient comfort. The décor was bright and colorful. Waiting lounges were filled with books, games, puzzles, reading areas, and snack machines. A photo on the wall showed young patients sitting on horses. The specialty hospital had a history of ensuring that kids were able to enjoy normal childhood experiences despite long inpatient stays. We transferred all of Cody's care to Gillette.

She was measured for a new back brace, ankle braces, and now a platform brace. Cody had to be strapped into the padded platform at night and sleep on her back. She was taught to line up Velcro straps to hold her legs in place. It was unimaginable to me that anyone could adjust to such restriction, but Cody adapted to sleeping in the frame without a problem.

At almost nine, Cody was nearing the appropriate age for the first of five spine surgeries to address the scoliosis that was crushing her lungs and displacing her heart. The body brace she'd worn for three years had allowed Cody to delay the serious surgical procedure presumably without further damage to her heart or compromising her lung capacity. Doctors estimated that the final surgery, a full spinal fusion, could be done once she gained ninety percent of her height, around age eleven or twelve. We'd hear more about these serious procedures over the next year. But first, Cody's legs needed straightening, and she realized she had no choice about it. She'd still be able to attend a summer school session and go to camp for twelve days before surgery. I promised to make sure she had a fun summer no matter what.

Her only comment was, "Doctors are stupid."

When I mentioned the operation that evening, Cody said, "*Look*, Mom, I don't want to discuss it. I'm going to have a nice week without seeing any doctors."

Pictures arrived in the mail from Tad's mother. She and Becky had driven Tad to the Abbey of the Genesee in New York where he was now a Trappist monk. Tad's head was shaved in a crew cut, his beard and mustache were trimmed close, and he wore a long white robe with a belt at the waist.

As we watched *That's Incredible* on television that night, the show ended with an invitation to "write in with your own incredible stories." Cody said, "We should send our names in."

I asked her what incredible thing we knew about. She turned both hands palms up and said, "My dad's in a monastery!"

With Dennis's heavy work schedule, Cody and I spent most of our time together without him that summer. I fixed breakfast; she fussed about what to wear. A bus picked her up for summer school. I painted while she was gone. Painting, exhibiting, and selling my artwork was now my only job. Most afternoons when Cody was dropped off, we talked about her day and sometimes watched *General Hospital* together. She kept her eye on the clock for when her next-door-neighbor friend Julie was due home. Often, Cody and her friends circled the block in a parade of toys on wheels while I worked in the garden. She allowed little kids to sit on her lap for rides in her wheelchair. I brought out drinks, crayons, and paper, or helped Cody onto the porch. When Dennis was home, he threw a Nerf football around with Cody in the evening, or we walked around the block with the dogs.

The night before Cody left for camp I read aloud as she got ready for bed. After prayers, she wanted me to tell the "Emmy story." The Emmy story was about the time Tad took a hot bath and stretched out on the bed before getting dressed. Our cat Emmy raced in, jumped onto the bed, bit Tad on the penis and raced away as Tad howled in pain. Cody laughed hard imagining Emmy's sneak attack. I used that story often when Cody was in the hospital to take her mind off the insertion of an IV, or with other unpleasant medical procedures such as blood draws or shots. She couldn't help laughing if I said, "Hey, babe, remember how Emmy bit Tad you-know-where?"

Cody spent the next twelve days at a summer camp for children with disabilities. Cabins were wheelchair accessible, and there was swimming, boating, and horseback riding. The counselors were comfortable working with kids with many types of handicaps. The staff included a doctor and a nurse.

Cody cried all morning and half the drive to camp, saying she'd changed her mind and didn't want to go. I promised she could call and I'd pick her up if she hated it after giving it a try for a few days. A half hour from camp, Cody announced, "Now, I'm excited."

Counselors greeted her with hugs and immediately involved her in a crafts project with other campers. She waved a casual goodbye when we drove away.

Dennis left for San Francisco and I was alone with the dogs. I was adjusting to Dennis's absences, but I missed daily contact with Cody, her sweet disposition, and wry sense of humor. I briefly considered driving to her camp for a surprise visit.

When she came home from camp, she had a bad cold that hung on so long that her surgery was postponed until August. Cody was pleased with the reprieve. The timing was serendipitous in that she could join me for an art opening where I sold some paintings.

Dennis came home in time for me to take an unplanned trip to Pittsburgh when my mother needed emergency surgery for a burst appendix. During the week I was there, I told Dad about the panic attacks I'd been having for two years. He told me Mom had panic attacks throughout her pregnancy with me. With this new information I decided to schedule an appointment with a psychotherapist when I returned to Minneapolis. But the night I came home, my brother Charlie called.

He had spoken to the man who, two years before, had the vision about Cody, the stream, and Jesus. He told Charlie, "Cody and her operation will be fine, but your sister and her husband need prayers. Your sister has been down on herself recently. She doesn't realize that God wants to work through her to help others. She should be open to the Lord with expectancy for him to use her in a wonderful way."

I felt waves of angel shivers as I listened to my brother deliver what sounded like a telegram from God. I told Charlie about my anxiety attacks. Right then he prayed for healing of my panic attacks and any inner memories that caused pain. He told me, "Exercise faith. Trust Jesus, even if you feel bad. Don't trust bad feelings. You can cancel that therapy appointment; you won't need it." Charlie was right. I never had another anxiety attack. *Thank God.*

Cody's surgeon said he'd had to break the bone above the knee in both of her legs to straighten them. The pins he placed in the bones could be removed after the fractures healed. Cody remained lying on her back for several weeks. We read books, listened to music, and hung around with the dogs. She didn't complain during the weeks of restriction, other than to say it was boring. Her one diversion was when friends invited us to spend Cody's ninth birthday at their lake house. Dennis and I slid her onto the backseat of the car in her sleep frame and secured the platform with seatbelts for the drive to the lake. Cody was able to breathe fresh air and ride on a pontoon boat. By the time school started, she was able to sit with her leg casts resting on the raised foot pedals of her wheelchair.

Cody was transferred to Hiawatha Elementary because Seward School did not have an accessible fourth grade classroom. The school district recommended half days at a "special" school that was equipped to assist with physical and occupational therapy. This proposition was tempting under the circumstances. We had learned too late that Cody's third grade teacher resented being forced to deal with a child in a wheelchair for the first time just as her teaching career was ending. She had placed Cody in a back corner, hadn't given her assignments with the rest of the class, and never told us when Cody had trouble keeping up with other students.

Dennis and I wanted Cody to have a more successful school experience, but we didn't want to go backwards in our quest for her to receive a mainstream education. Teachers in the special school were kindhearted people who understood disability, and since Cody's legs were in casts as the school year started, we agreed to the split-day arrangement.

When the time came to remove the pins in Cody's thighbones, no anesthesia was required, so the procedure was done in the outpatient clinic at Gillette. Dennis and I stood on either side, holding Cody's hands as the doctor prepared to remove the first pin, which looked more like a big nail. I blurred my eyes and looked into Cody's face so that I didn't focus on the tugging and parting of her flesh, or the trickle of blood coming from the open hole.

Dennis looked directly at the procedure and promptly fainted. As his body dropped away from the gurney where Cody lay, his backward fall was partly cushioned by a laundry bin. Cody grabbed my head with both of her strong arms and slammed my face into her chest, saying, "Don't faint, Mom! Don't faint!"

The doctor, nurses, and aides immediately left Cody, surrounded Dennis, and lifted him by his arms and legs onto a nearby exam table. I tried to speak, but my voice was muffled in Cody's clothing and body brace as she clamped down on my head. I spoke into her sweater, "Cody, let me up. I won't faint."

Cody released my head but hung onto my hands. Dennis remained supine until after the pins were removed. "Poor Daddy!" Cody said.

One of the kids at Cody's special school was a friend she met at summer camp. Rachel was in a wheelchair due to cerebral palsy (CP). Her movement was slow but CP didn't affect her speech. She and Cody joined Girl Scouts together. Rachel became a regular visitor at our house. She stayed overnight on a chair that unfolded to a single bed next to Cody's bed. When she couldn't wait any longer for Rachel to wake up in the morning, Cody folded the bed, with Rachel still in it. Rachel woke up laughing. The girls pulled pranks and tried new things together. They once made organic soil with coffee grounds and garbage for a school project and put the smelly mixture inside the heat vent in Cody's bedroom to hurry the process along.

Because Cody missed so many school days due to colds that fall, the school assessment team decided to consider that year a combination of grades three and four. Cody coughed so hard at one point that I said, "I'm sorry you're so sick. I feel like a bad mother."

Cody responded with a disapproving sniff, "That's ridiculous. No mother is perfect, not you, not your mother, not your grandmother."

At the December clinic appointment the urologist showed Cody a film to teach her how to use a catheter. That night at home, she demonstrated what she learned. She sat on the floor, pulled her legs apart, and guided a latex catheter by feel alone into her urethra to drain her bladder. I marveled that she was able to do it. I showered her with compliments.

This new skill offered valuable independence. Cody had never been able to be away for more than a few hours from someone who knew how to cath her. She was already adept at using a slider board to transfer to and from her chair and other similar height surfaces. She could roll from her chair onto a bed and pull herself back into her wheelchair. Now that she could cath herself, all she needed was a private place and a sink to wash her hands. This achievement was a major turning point in Cody's self-reliance. She beamed at her accomplishment.

However, somber news had come from an orthopedic surgeon at the same appointment. Cody was about to enter her "growth spurt." The time had come to plan five spine surgeries. The first would be the follow-ing summer, when a metal Harrington rod would be implanted along one side of her spine, attached to vertebrae at each end by metal wires and ratchets. Six months later, the rod would be lengthened at each end to allow her continued growth.

Six months after that, a second rod would be installed on the other side of her spine, to be lengthened in six more months. Two years after the first rod was implanted, Cody's spine would be permanently fused. The final operation would occur the summer Cody turned twelve. Once her spine was fused, she could not grow any taller.

Five operations over the next two years sounded daunting. Dennis and I agreed with Cody not to think about it until after Christmas. We were going east for the holidays. Cody was going to visit "Daddy Tad" in the monastery.

Chapter 9

Mainstream Fusion

TAD WAS ALLOWED a two-night visit with Cody, so I wanted to arrive at the Abbey of the Genesee as early as possible the first day. At 3:30 in the morning, wearing new Christmas sweaters that Tad's mother knitted for each of us, Dennis, Cody, and I left in a rental car from Becky and Robert's house in Bucks County. Cody and her little cousin Maia had taken a warm bath together and gone to sleep early the night before. Snowflakes bounced off the windshield as we drove in the dark. Cody slept in the backseat, wrapped in a blanket for most of the five-and-a-half-hour drive into western New York State.

The aroma of fresh-baked bread filled the crisp air at the monastery. Tad stood in the morning sunshine, wearing a woolen jacket over a long white monk's robe. He waved us toward a parking area in front of the guesthouse. Greeting us with hugs, he helped unload Cody's wheelchair. He pushed Cody up the walk to our accommodations while asking questions about people and events in the "outside world."

The guest mansion was an attractive old home with many bedrooms. The linens were white, the ceilings were high, and the décor was simple but elegant. There were no other inhabitants during our stay. Tad explained that he was wearing his monk's robe because he was due at church shortly after our arrival. Monks gathered six times a day at specific intervals, starting at 2:25 a.m., to sing and pray. Tad otherwise wore regular street clothes because the Abbey was a working monastery. Like each of the monks, he had assigned chores, including bread-baking. Public demand for the delicious Monk's Bread was constant. We ate lots of it during our visit.

Both mornings before five o'clock, we wheeled Cody across the yard to the Abbey church where monks sang and prayed at a service called lauds. In a chapel lit only with candles, a few dozen monks sat or stood in rows on each side of an altar. The area for guest seating was in the back behind a wooden rail. The chorus of men's voices was hypnotic. Cody was too sleepy that early to express interest in the surroundings; she was just happy to see Tad. The entire monastic environment, even outside the chapel, was quiet. The brothers we met smiled and spoke in low tones, telling Cody they'd heard so much about her.

Between Tad's regular duties and prayer times, he played with Cody and told us about life as a Trappist monk. He found a closet to fall out of for her entertainment and joined us in the evening to tuck in Cody and sing bedtime songs. We harmonized and repeated the chorus of "Circle Game" as she drifted to sleep.

After Cody was in bed the second evening, Tad told me that, although he felt at peace in the contemplative community, he thought perhaps he was meant for a more active ministry. I didn't try to sway his thinking either way, but I privately hoped he'd decide to leave the monastery so Cody could see him more often.

Tad waved as we drove away from the monastery the following day. Cody sobbed, "I want my daddy." She called Tad "Daddy" whenever she missed him. Dennis hugged her while I drove. The weather was bitter cold. We reached Pittsburgh around midnight with gifts of Monk's Bread for my parents. Dad cooked a delicious late dinner for us. Cody talked excitedly about seeing Maia and visiting Tad at the Abbey. We flew home the next day to find weather even colder in Minneapolis—minus twenty-six degrees with a windchill of seventy below.

Keeping Cody's wheelchair ramp clear of snow was a challenge every winter. Neighboring sidewalks were rarely shoveled well enough for a wheelchair to pass. The metal on Cody's chair was often ice-cold to the touch.

That winter, Cody had a couple of what I considered "typical" health-related procedures for a child of nine, things not connected to her disability. That "normal" quality made them seem, in some ways, easier. The ear, nose, and throat consult determined that Cody's frequent colds were probably due to enlarged adenoids. These were removed at Gillette Hospital. Then, a tooth was extracted in preparation for braces.

While recovering from her pulled tooth, Cody and I were sitting with the dogs in Cody's bedroom, having one of our chats about this and that. I sat on the floor with Milka in my lap. Sadie sat on the bed with her snout a few inches from Cody's face as she ate a bowl of ice cream. Used to such close attention from Sadie, Cody kept eating without pause and smacked her lips with relish at each spoonful.

"Hey, Mom, I had an idea. Wouldn't it be funny to have dog court? Characters in the courtroom would be cans of dog food that argue for the privilege of being eaten by Sadie." Cody described various details of her canine courtroom drama, laughing at each detail she imagined. Sadie leaned closer as her eyes followed the spoon from bowl to mouth. Cody finished her last bit of ice cream and sighed, "That would be funny . . . and that's the truth, the whole truth."

Sadie cleaned the bowl and spoon.

Our little beagle had an insatiable appetite. The day after Easter, she devoured all the candy in Cody's Easter basket. Cody was crestfallen to lose her entire stash of sweets, so I went to Target and came home with new candy. She said sincerely, "Thank you very much, Mom. I wish I could do something for you—like take out the trash."

This was a chore Cody could not do because of the logistics of our back steps, but I knew she genuinely wished she could. Cody reached into her basket, held out her favorite candy bar and offered, "Would you like to split this with me?"

I said, "No, thank you, sweetie," and had to smile at how relieved she looked.

Cody's stories and poems from her earliest school years were often about her dogs, with descriptions of dog behavior. She shared my abhorrence for animal cruelty and came with me to meetings held by animal protection organizations. Cody hand-lettered a protest sign that said *Don't Hurt Animals*. Such interests led to my becoming a vegetarian and a board member of Animal Rights Coalition (ARC). I was honest with Cody about sources of food. I explained that pork, bacon, and ham were other words for parts of a dead pig, and made similar explanations about beef, veal, and steak. Cody decided, "I don't want to eat animals anymore."

On the phone she told her friend Rachel, "Rach! Do you know what chicken really is? It's chickens! They're *killed* and made into *food!*"

Dennis's activism was ignited in his role as part of a group advocating for education and accessibility rights for people with handicaps. The information he learned reinforced our resolve to return Cody full time to a regular school. Her school day was still divided between Hiawatha Elementary and the Dowling School for kids with disabilities. So much emphasis was placed on activities related to disabilities or behavioral problems with other children that the educational aspects of the half day at Dowling appeared secondary.

School system officials announced their intent to start a "formal" mainstreaming program, touting it as a "progressive" project. The plan sounded promising, at first. However, not a single child in a wheelchair in the entire district was to be placed full time in a regular school. A lengthy startup process included evaluations and "readiness preparation." Assessment folks at Dowling were supposed to decide when kids like Cody were "ready" for a regular school.

At the periodic review of Cody's individual educational plan (IEP), Dennis and I expressed our frustration. Dennis reminded administrators that the idea of mainstreaming was to bring students with disabilities *into* the mainstream, not separate them from other students.

IEP meetings were commonly held in a room with long tables. A child's parents sat on one side. As many as six to ten school representatives sat on the other side, maintaining that they knew best for the child. In light of a venue designed to intimidate, it was easy to guess why so few parents came forward to insist on a fully accessible education for their kids.

Dennis and I looked across the table and stated in no uncertain terms that we wanted our daughter in a regular school, full time. Our uphill struggle continued.

Cody created two paintings for the annual International Art Show by Disabled Artists at Sister Kenny Institute in Minneapolis. The artists' opening in April included wine, cheese, and a live band. The exhibit featured paintings by artists from thirteen countries. Cody had been to many of my art openings, but this time she was in the spotlight. She was blasé about the whole event but had a huge smile in the photo Dennis took of her in front of her paintings.

By the end of the school year we found a small two-bedroom bungalow on one level, only thirteen blocks away. The house needed work, but I could do most of the repairs and projects myself. I removed three steps from the driveway up to the fenced-in backyard to make the house wheelchair accessible from the street. Dennis helped dig out the area for a cement sidewalk that wound through the yard, around the side of the house, and up to a wooden ramp to the front door. Adjusted gate latches allowed Cody to come and go without assistance. She took Milka outside for walks around the block that summer. The cockapoo accompanied Cody wherever she wheeled. She sat patiently if Cody stopped to daydream or watch for neighborhood friends. Milka was so attentive that Cody called the dog her "little mother."

The best part of the new neighborhood was our neighbors. The family in the house across the back alley had five pretty little girls, each two years apart. The oldest was a year younger than Cody. We'd seen the Newberg family a few times at St. Albert's before we moved. Art and his wife Robbie were warm, friendly people. Cody played with all five girls. Several families nearby belonged to St. Albert's. Neighbors gathered regularly for potlucks and parties.

Dennis missed Cody's first spine surgery to implant a Harrington rod due to a trip he took to Turkey and England for several weeks. Tad came to be with Cody for her surgery. He had left the monastery to join a faith community in New York City that helped runaway youth.

Tad and I said a prayer with Cody as she was taken into the operating room. She emerged from the recovery room with a bandaged incision that went from the back of her neck down the entire length of her spine.

She was wide-awake by dinnertime, eating Jell-O and sipping ginger ale through a straw. Tad spent the night on a cot next to Cody's hospital bed.

She shut her eyes and asked him to sing. After he finished four verses of "Circle Game," she reached for his hand. "Sing it again." When snorty breathing noises indicated that Cody was finally asleep, Tad leaned forward to kiss her cheek. She mumbled, "Hey! Keep singing."

Cody sat up in her wheelchair the next day. Her straight posture was supported by a newly formed plastic brace around her torso. Trying to move her head up and down, she said she felt stiff. She wheeled forward cautiously. "I'm afraid to move like normal. I'm afraid I'll break."

"The doctor said you won't break," I reminded her. "You just can't ride a horse or go on rough amusement park rides. He says your back is actually stronger than before."

Cody adapted to the new position of her spine within a day of being home from the hospital. She told Rachel, "I like being straight. I feel tall. I don't lean anymore when I sit up."

The scar itched "like crazy." Cody was happy when I finally snipped and removed the stitches in time for her tenth birthday, which was spent driving to Chicago for my brother Billy's wedding. Charlie, my oldest brother and prayer-for-a-miracle partner, came from Missouri with his wife Edie and their two kids. Julie was a year older than Cody. The cousins had been together only briefly on a few occasions but they bonded naturally. Julie sat near Cody or played with her on the floor. Five-year-old Zachary was a bundle of energy. Cody was captivated and laughed as "Little Zachie" wrestled with his dad. The girls giggled like best friends as Julie braided Cody's hair and added ribbons for the ceremony. They passed out programs and welcomed the wedding guests.

School administrators again touted the new "mainstreaming" program at a planning meeting before Cody started a full year of fourth grade. The only thing new, as far as we could see, was that Cody's school day was split between the school for kids with disabilities and the now "official" mainstream location, Anderson.

Our argument continued in favor of placing Cody full time at Anderson, but we didn't press hard in light of her recent back surgery. We decided a more protective environment for part of the day might be safer for the moment. The woman in charge of the mainstreaming initiative tried to convince us that this model already was a formal mainstreaming program. We wanted to believe her.

The Anderson school administrator informed parents in a letter that Cody and any other "handicapped guests" would not start school until three weeks into the school year. The purpose of the delay was so teachers had "time to get to know the other students" first. Dennis wrote a blistering response to school officials protesting the three-week start delay and objecting to the term "guests" for mainstreamed children. He pointed out that there was no valid reason for teachers to "get to know" other students first or deprive mainstreamed children from the unique experience of starting school with the rest of their class.

Cody was still not challenged academically under the divided-day arrangement. Nor was there a protective advantage for Cody because her back incision healed quickly. Transport time alone between the two schools wasted a chunk of every day. On the other hand, Cody was enjoying school. Her friend Rachel was also at Dowling and Cody liked helping other kids with things she could already do well. Rather than make a change during the school year, Dennis and I decided to focus on ensuring that Cody was *truly* mainstreamed next year when she'd start fifth grade.

Dennis was in Massachusetts when a research paper he wrote about unemployment received wide media attention. Major news networks, public radio, and *USA Today* interviewed him. Cody and I proudly called our friends and relatives with the news that he was on the front page of the *Wall Street Journal*.

Cody and I were sick in bed with chest colds the week Dennis was gone. She coughed especially hard one night and had a bloody nose at 2:00 a.m. She climbed into my bed and the dogs curled up with us. We spent so much time feeling miserable that week; we pretended to have a contest about who was sicker. I was winning until the nosebleed. Cody said, "Now we're even."

We chatted in the dark. Cody was concerned about Tad's youngest brother. Grandma Cornell had told her by phone that Michael was diagnosed with dyslexia. Cody knew from friends at school that people with dyslexia had trouble reading. She said, "Poor Michael, poor Michael. I'm going to read to Uncle Michael when we visit at Christmas."

She asked, "Mom, I don't want to be mean, but could you give me back the orange cup I made for you at camp, so I can give it to Uncle Michael for Christmas?"

I nodded yes as I had another coughing fit. Twice in the night, as I had coughing attacks, I felt Cody's hand rest on my back and heard her whisper prayers for me.

My ARC friend, Sam, phoned one evening to tell me about a severely neglected dog. For months the owner kept the small dog tied outside, leaving him on weekends without food or water. A neighbor, fearful of the owner and unable to convince any humane society to intervene, kidnapped the dog and brought him to Sam. "No one will adopt him," Sam told me. "His hair is so matted I can't see his eyes. I think he's a cockapoo like Milka. Will you cut his hair?"

Cody was at school when Sam arrived the next morning and handed me what looked like a pile of tangled, dusty black wool. I lay the raggedy dog on newspapers spread on the dining room table. He held still as I examined him. Hair twisted close to his skin was embedded with twigs and dirt. He was unable to stretch out his legs due to matted hair knotted to his stomach. His toenails curled into his paw pads. I started clipping around his eyes so he could see. For hours, I cut away clump after clump, working closer to his skin. His eyes stayed on my face as I told him over and over what a good boy he was.

When Cody came home from school, she took over, saying soothing things and stroking his tiny body. She helped bathe him, and we clipped knots of hair until Dennis came home from work. The three of us worked into the evening to trim the tender areas.

When we were done, the pile of hair cut away was larger than the dog himself. Once on the floor he stood still for a moment and endured curious sniffing from Milka and Sadie. Like an unwinding spring, he ran with increasing speed through the house, from the enclosed front porch into the living room, dining room, kitchen, and back again. We took him out to the backyard where he ran around the perimeter of the fence. Cody crooned, "Aww, poor little sweetie."

Our vet treated the little dog for fleas and worms and neutered him in preparation for adoption. He weighed in at eight pounds. Each day after school, Cody and I walked him to a nearby park and let him off the leash to run. He kept his eyes on us as he ran in widening circles around the baseball diamond and through the trees. He ran back past us after each circle and took off again.

Even Dennis, who never did share our devotion to dogs, thought Dan was adorable. We started calling him Dan in homage to Father Dan from St. Albert's. I don't think Father Dan was particularly flattered, but we considered it a compliment.

By Christmastime our family was in agreement. We didn't want to find another home for Dan. He was home with us. Cody said, "Sadie is your dog, Mom. Milka is Dad's dog, and now, Dan is *MY* dog." We flew east again for the holidays, but Cody said the best part of that Christmas was adopting Dan.

Cody sailed through her second spine surgery in January to lengthen the metal Harrington rod put there the previous summer. She was allowed to arrive at the hospital the morning of surgery and go home as soon as she recovered from anesthesia. The incision was only a few inches at each end of her spine to allow for the extension of the rod. Cody was in high spirits to have accomplished such a serious operation without an overnight stay.

In March, I started a half-time job working with lawyers. I was home each day in time to paint and help Cody with homework after school. Dennis's academic research work continued to receive media attention and involve regular travel. Cody and I painted or watched television together in the evenings. She transferred onto the couch next to the dogs and me while we watched the entire *Thornbirds* series about a ranch family in Australia. Cody developed a crush on its star, Richard Chamberlain. She begged, "Can we please go to California to meet him?"

She sent away for his picture and hung it in her room with other favorites: Ricky Schroeder and Michael Jackson. She wanted to find a way to meet Michael Jackson, too. In a serious voice Cody said, "He's cool, Mom. He's nice to people in wheelchairs."

Rachel stayed overnight every couple of weeks and sometimes on school nights. The girls stayed up late reading movie magazines and planning strategies for contacting famous people. They called television stations and scanned phone books.

Cody had tried the phone book technique some years earlier when she found out that Mr. Rogers of *Mr. Rogers Neighborhood* lived in Pittsburgh. On a visit with my parents, she'd called every Rogers in the Pittsburgh phone book. There was only one "F." Rogers. Cody was full of expectation when a woman answered the phone. Cody asked, "Is Mr. Rogers there?"

"Not the Mr. Rogers you want, honey."

Not deterred, Cody reminded me, "Mom, lots of famous people live in Minnesota." She and Rachel were convinced that they would "at least" contact a member of The Jets.

Cody sold two paintings in the Sister Kenny art show that spring. Instead of rainbows and clouds, her new images were of flying saucers and maps. Each piece sold for twenty-five dollars the night of the opening.

That summer, Cody and the neighborhood girls performed musical theater in our garage. Scenes from *Annie* were drawn in crayon on the inside garage walls. Cody wore a curly orange wig for the title role. Our neighborhood was full of little girls who were perfect fits for a play about kids in an orphanage. They sang, *"It's a hard knock life for us . . ."*

Refreshments were served and homemade programs were passed out. Neighbor families sat in lawn chairs in our driveway to watch the performances.

Cody was reluctant to leave the neighborhood fun to go to camp. After her second day, I received a letter begging me to bring her home, signed with a picture of a frowning face and the words, "This is me." Alarmed that she sounded so miserable, I called camp as soon as I read the letter. Cody came to the phone with a cheery, "Hi, Mom, what's up?"

"Well, I got your letter. You sounded homesick."

"Yeah, I was. But I'm having fun now."

"Okay then."

Tad came to Minneapolis in time to pick up Cody from camp. He wanted to see her before going to Rome for a year to study at a Dominican university. He joined the cast of the girl's garage production of *Annie* in the role of Daddy Warbucks for two performances. And, at Cody's request, he fell out of the closet several times to entertain her girlfriends.

In July an intestinal virus kept me from being with Cody for her third spine surgery. Dennis stayed with her the only night she spent at Gillette Hospital. The long surgery to install the second Harrington rod went smoothly. But, eight days later, Cody's shunt broke down. Her neurosurgeon directed us to the emergency room at St. Paul Children's Hospital.

I was tense as we waited for Cody to be taken into brain surgery. I wondered why her shunt broke down so soon after a major operation. Did the long hours under anesthesia for her back surgery cause excess fluid pressure in her shunt? She lay on the gurney with her hand holding a towel to shield her eyes from ceiling lights. Trying to ignore the pain in her head, Cody said, "I want to do something fun for my eleventh birthday."

We talked about a slumber party until she was wheeled to the operating room. She came out of recovery with a puffy face and a long drop of dried Betadine on her neck. With incisions in four places, and one side of her head shaved in the back, she looked beat-up. As Cody was wheeled back to her room, I took her hand and said, "Hi, babe," in a sympathetic mom voice.

She opened her eyes and said, "I want to rent the movie *Fame* for my birthday. How many girls can I invite to spend the night?"

In August, at a school meeting three days before Cody turned eleven, administrators reviewed Cody's academic assessment test scores from the previous spring. Her lowest score was in math: slightly below fourth grade level. Her highest was in reading: above sixth grade level. Dennis and I were immovable in our decision that Cody start fifth grade full time in a regular school.

A school official warned that Cody would miss the benefits provided at Dowling, which their report described as help with: (1) completing academic tasks, (2) physical therapy and independent living skills, and (3) increasing peer socialization.

I took issue with the necessity of *any* of the three items. (1) Rather than give Cody academic work, Dowling had provided her with a place to do the homework assigned during the half day she spent at Anderson. (2) After she fell while in her stander the first year at Dowling, Cody refused to use it anymore. Physical therapy was now mainly stretching exercises. I explained that those were more appropriately done at home, as well. (3) There was no evidence that a half day at Dowling enhanced her peer socialization. In fact, pulling her away from Anderson in the middle of the day made it hard for Cody to develop relationships with non-disabled kids. Dennis and I reasserted that Cody would not go back to Dowling for *any* part of *any* day.

The woman in charge of the mainstreaming program looked alarmed when the Anderson principal endorsed our decision. She looked perplexed as it sunk in that Cody was actually about to be mainstreamed. Noticing her expression Dennis asked gently, "Wasn't this the goal of your program in the first place?"

"Well, yes, but . . ." Her voice trailed off.

Cody became the first child in a wheelchair in the Minneapolis School District Mainstreaming Project to be fully mainstreamed. I noticed a difference immediately. School subjects stimulated her. She brought home stories and new ideas every day. I heard her tell Rachel, "It's better at my new school."

After Cody's first month at Anderson, the school district sent a Dowling assessment team to evaluate her progress. The report included comments about her physical skills and interactions with others, concluding: "Cody is comfortable talking about her physical handicap and has a positive self-image. When other students approach her to push her wheelchair for her, she tells them she can push herself."

I supposed that meant she had assimilated successfully. But there were other things about her life in the new school that said much more to me. Cody was studious about completing her homework. And she was a blossoming preteen. She asked my advice about a boy in her class. "He's so cute. How can I talk to him? What should I say?"

She didn't take the advice I suggested, but I was touched that she asked.

Sadie's hind legs stopped working that fall. She strained to drag herself around by her front legs. Our dear old beagle had slipped a disc. The vet said a long back surgery might not help at her age. Even if it did, any improvement would be slight. Dennis carried her to the yard and back in the mornings. Cody caressed her and spoke soothingly to her. There was no change after ten days of treatment and medication, but Sadie never complained.

I cried when I told my parents. Mom said a prayer for Sadie on the phone. Dad said, "You've had a great thing in Sadie but, if I were her, I'd want you to pull the plug once my life wasn't comfortable. There's no point in extending her discomfort or your family's stress."

I knew what I had to do. I cried with Cody that night when I explained it to her. The next day, we took Sadie to the vet. Cody chose not to be in the room with her beloved friend as she died. I stroked my beagle's velvety face as she quietly slipped away. Cody sobbed in the waiting room and hugged Dennis. She wrote in her journal, "This was the saddest day of my life."

In January, the second Harrington rod was lengthened in preparation for the full spinal fusion in August. Tad planned to leave Italy to be with Cody for the final surgery. Dennis was away in England for several weeks early in the summer, and I was asked to write a review of a conference in London only the week before Cody's operation. Given the timing, I invited Cody to come on the trip with me. She said, "I'll think about it."

She didn't think long before politely declining my invitation. Sounding so levelheaded and mature, she explained that she didn't want to be away from home right before a big surgery.

As I helped Cody pack for camp, she began to cry. I asked what was wrong. Her voice quivered. "What would happen to me if Dad and you both died while I was at camp?"

"I'm sure Robbie would take care of you until my parents got here."
I thought of our neighbor Robbie as an ideal mother.

Cody asked, "How do you know that?"

I said, "We'll call and ask her."

Robbie listened as I described Cody's concern, and said, "Of course
we'd keep Cody."

I told Cody, "Robbie says she would keep you." In an awkward attempt
to lighten the mood, I added, "She'd even adopt you."

Robbie immediately said, "Yes, I would adopt Cody."

"Are you kidding?" I sputtered, "You already have five daughters!"

Robbie repeated, "Yes, I really would adopt Cody."

Tears stung my eyes. I knew Robbie understood the ramifications of her
words. I stumbled through a thank you, but knew of no adequate way to
express my gratitude to her for giving Cody and me such peace of mind.

Later, Cody and I talked more about Robbie's amazing offer. Cody's eyes
sparkled as she said how much fun it would be to have five little sisters.

"Hey, wait a minute, kiddo." I said, "We're not dead yet!"

Cody giggled and said, "Oh, yeah!"

Cody sent me a cheerful letter from camp with a happy face that said,
"This is me, today," and a sad face that said, "This was me, yesterday."

When I picked her up, she said, "Robbie and four Newberg girls visited
me. And Robin was the best counselor I ever had. If she's there next year, I
want to go back for sure."

Like each summer, Cody had been gone twelve days. But this time,
she looked older to me. Her face appeared thinner, her cheekbones more
defined. I couldn't put my finger on the difference, but Cody seemed less
a little girl and more like a young woman. During the next few weeks, she
wrote several letters to Robin and burst into tears a few times, missing her
so much. She talked on about how much fun and how "cool" Robin was.

I remembered a camp counselor I adored at thirteen. However, despite
the powerful emotion I'd felt, it never occurred to me to mention it to my
mother. I was grateful that Cody, at almost twelve, still told me about such
feelings. She took out her diary to write about Robin and said, "I may want
this to be private for a few years, Mom. You can read it when I grow up."

Cody began watching TV and didn't write in her diary that night. Even so, I was proud of her impulse to do it.

Four weeks before the spinal fusion, Cody began to feel scared. I tried to distract her with birthday plans but found it hard to deal with her fears when they were so close to my own. We reminded each other that her friend Brian had no problems with his spine fusion.

Cody said, "I want Uncle Charlie and his friends to pray for me again. Last time, it started my foot moving. Maybe this time I'll be able to walk. That's a miracle I would love."

I said a prayer right then with Cody. "Please, God, make this surgery quick, successful, and for Cody not to have to undergo anything so serious again. In Jesus' name, amen."

Cody said, "It would be so great to walk. I'd love to surprise Dennis by meeting him at the airport walking."

By phone, Charlie agreed to initiate requests with prayer groups for God to work through Cody's doctors and to take away our fears about the huge surgery.

I told Cody, "Charlie said he believes you'll be healed some day."

She said, "If Uncle Charlie says so, then it's true."

Cody called me to her room that night to ask if I could see her right foot move. I felt tugging in her foot, but I wasn't sure. I remembered how young she was when I began prayers for a miracle so that her life wasn't in danger. Now, again, I prayed for faith.

The battle was on between faith and fear. I was scared for my daughter and I didn't want her to know it. After she was asleep, I called Father Dan. I told him I was scared about the coming fusion surgery. I told him I thought I was handling Cody okay, but not me.

Despite the late hour, Dan said, "I'll be right over." He showed up with two loaves of bread and a booklet of prayers. He said, "Everyone at church knows Cody; she has an effect on everyone." He drank my awful instant coffee and listened to my worries that night until we were both laughing and I felt much better.

Cody was happy to have all three parents with her as she was wheeled into the operating room. The spine fusion operation took many hours, but "everything went perfectly." Tad, Dennis, and I surrounded Cody when she came back from the recovery room. The effects of anesthesia wore off quickly. We all joked around and felt great relief. But within an hour of our happy talk, Cody became lethargic and her eyes showed signs of intracranial pressure. I asked the nurse to call a neurosurgeon. By the time the physician on call arrived, Cody was still and hard to rouse. The doctor took a quick look at her and said she looked fine to him, adding, "It's normal to be groggy like this after a big surgery."

"No, it's not normal for her," I said, "She was awake and chirpy two hours ago."

I could see by his facial expression that I wasn't getting through to this doctor. He'd never seen Cody before. He had a thick foreign accent; I suspected a language barrier. I tried again to explain clearly what was happening to Cody. He shrugged me off and started to leave. My voice shook as I shouted, "Wait!"

Dennis took over. "Listen, our daughter is not her normal postoperative self."

He continued to argue with the doctor. I retreated to the bathroom next to Cody's bed. I wanted to scream in frustration. I shut the door, had an angry cry for a few seconds, splashed water on my face, dried off with paper towels, and went back out. Now Tad was facing the physician. His voice rose as he stressed, "Cody could *die* here!"

I looked straight into the doctor's eyes and spoke slowly. "Look. Our child is in trouble; she needs surgery now. We've been told by her regular neurosurgeon that we should not wait when she has these symptoms. She could stop breathing!"

The physician was frustrated and flustered. He waved his arm and gestured to a nurse passing in the hall to come into the room. He asked her, "What has gone on with this patient?"

The nurse confirmed that Cody had been fine right after surgery. "She was talking and laughing. She wasn't like this."

The doctor's demeanor changed instantly. He arranged immediate neurosurgery. Tad, Dennis, and I maintained our vigil around Cody's bed. My head throbbed with a sudden migraine as she was wheeled into the operating room.

The doctor told us later that he found debris in the shunt tubing; the valve had stopped working. Keeping his eyes on a chart, he said, "She'll be fine now."

Cody was awake and crunching ice chips within two hours, and discharged the next morning. Her twelfth birthday was celebrated days later with a houseful of friends. A baseball cap helped cover her missing hair. Dan curled in Cody's lap and Milka rested her head on a wheelchair foot pedal while Cody opened gifts and thanked each giver.

Cody still went from place to place in a wheelchair, had metal rods in her spine and a shunt in her brain. But she was alive, happy, and home with her family. I was grateful. I thought, *What is the exact definition of a miracle?*

Chapter 10

Beaches

A NINE-DAY RETREAT in a large vacation house in Clearwater, Florida, over Thanksgiving was the longest time Cody had ever spent with my family. Fourteen of us came together to celebrate my parents' fiftieth wedding anniversary. The weather was chilly and windy, the sun bright. Cody wore sweatpants and a T-shirt the first morning and sat in the sand next to my father and mother. In the three months since her spinal fusion and shunt surgery, her hair hadn't grown out much. A floppy hat shaded her face as she collected seashells and watched gulls and pelicans swoop and dive toward the water. Cody's aunts and uncles sat in clusters on the sand or in beach chairs. Her cousins Julie and Zachary waded in the water.

As Cody transferred onto a bed to change her ib before lunch, she said, "Grandma is so protective of Grandpa. She always wants him covered up. She says, 'Gordon, you should wear a hat.' Really, if the man wanted to wear a hat, he would!"

Cody, Julie, and Zachary were the only kids in the group. Julie was already a young lady at thirteen. Zach had just turned seven. He was the life of the party. He was as energetic as Cody remembered him from their fun together two years before at my brother Billy's wedding. Now he told funnier stories. Julie teased him constantly. Cody laughed along, but kept her eye on Zach and came to his defense even as she was amused. Hearing jokes at his expense, Cody said, "Awww, Zachie," in the midst of a laugh.

Zach appreciated the alliance. He asked Cody if he could push her wheelchair "really" fast, and she let him. She smiled in delight as he raced her through the large rooms of the house and along the driveway and sidewalks. Weather was too cold for swimming, so the kids played Monster on the beach. They huddled together under blankets and screamed when my brother Charlie crept up on them.

The girls put on makeup to look beautiful for Thanksgiving dinner. Julie showed Cody how to apply eye shadow and mascara to enhance her eyes, and powder blush to make her cheeks rosy. The adults put together a fine holiday meal.

Zach finished eating and whispered to Cody, "Wanna go for a ride?"

She said, "Sure." Zach grabbed the wheelchair handles and pulled Cody away from the table. Older folks suggested that Zach settle down, but Cody loved every minute of the wild ride.

As the rest of us left the table, Julie turned on the stereo. Everyone began to move to the music. This was a family first. Each of us had a distinctive, if not peculiar, dance style. Billy spun on the living room floor with his feet in the air. Mom and Dad looked dapper, dancing in each other's arms. Edie and Charlie rocked with the jitterbug and the twist. The rest of us hopped around and gyrated. Cody was breathless with laughter as she boogied in her wheelchair. Her grandparents twirled and collapsed onto a lounge chair with Mom on Dad's lap.

Dad hugged Mom and said, "I'm still glad I married you."

We all cheered, clapped, and kept dancing. Mom moved to a seat in front of Cody and mimicked her movements by shaking her shoulders and waving her arms. Cody roared with laughter. After three or four lively songs, everyone flopped onto couches and chairs.

Cody looked around the room at her relatives and suggested that we say a prayer together. These were folks who'd been praying for her for all of her twelve years. My parents and brothers lived in four different states; this was the first time since Cody was five that my family was all in one place. Everyone obliged and gathered around, each putting a hand on Cody. One by one, they added prayers for her to be healed. Zach prayed last and ended his prayer, "Please make all pain leave Cody's body. Amen." He looked at Cody in faith-filled expectation and said, "Okay, stand up!"

Cody looked at her sweet young cousin with a loving smile and said,

"I can show you how I move my foot. I used to not be able to do that, but now I can."

She pulled off her sneaker and wiggled her left foot for Zach.

My brother Richard spent some part of every day chatting with Cody. He had always treated her more like a peer than a child. She enjoyed the feeling of respect. Cody told me, "I think your little brother is cute."

It sounded funny hearing Richard called my "little" brother. At almost six-three, he was the tallest in the family. Cody cried when he had to go back to work a few days sooner than the rest of us. She sobbed, "I love Uncle Richard. He's the little brother I never had."

Dennis left for Australia after Thanksgiving and came home a few days before Christmas. His mood was distant. He finally confessed that, after almost seven years of marriage, he wasn't sure he wanted to be a husband and father anymore.

Though not the first time he'd said something like that, I'd not seen it coming this time. After a marathon of talking and crying that night, I told Dennis that I didn't want to lose him and that Cody and I loved and needed him. I asked him to talk to Father Dan. The next day, Dennis began to cry when he told the priest about his feelings.

Cody appeared blasé at first when she learned that Dennis might move out, but later she cried and cried. I hugged her and told her how sorry I was and assured her that Dennis still loved her. I told her I didn't understand what was going on with him, but I promised I would never, ever leave her. Tears rolled down her cheeks as she said, "I don't want him to go. But I don't want him to stay just because of me."

I hated Dennis right then for the hurt Cody was feeling. I didn't know how to make her feel better. Each time she started to cry, I suggested she open a Christmas present. She liked that.

Tad came Christmas day for an overnight visit. He looked crestfallen hearing about our troubles and did his best to lift Cody's mood. He fell out of the closet a few times and played games with her. It was a difficult holiday. Rachel spent the night New Year's Eve. She and Cody went outside at midnight, yelled "Happy New Year" and banged saucepans.

Dennis didn't leave after all. Instead, we began sessions in January with a marriage counselor. We had lots of family conversations. We tried a self-esteem exercise at bedtime that I'd read about in a magazine. We told each other things we liked about the other.

Dennis said he appreciated my sense of humor, and he liked it that I didn't complain when I was sick. I told him how much I appreciated everything he did for Cody. We started to do the exercise with Cody at bedtime after saying prayers together. There was never a shortage of things to tell Cody that we liked about her. She liked that our family stayed together.

Cody was twelve when she took off her back brace for the last time. She'd worn the plastic contraption for seven years, every day and every night. The most recent versions of the brace had cutouts in the plastic for her developing breasts. In late February, six months after her spinal fusion, the orthopedic surgeon was satisfied that Cody's spine was healed. The brace was history. So too was the sleeping frame that had strapped her down every night.

After the appointment, Dennis and I took Cody out for a celebratory lunch, then to Target. Cody had a list of clothes she wanted to buy now that there were no more restrictions on the types of blouses or pants she could wear. No longer was she limited to smock-style tops, oversized loose shirts, and stretch pants. She now could consider form-fitting clothes, belts, V-neck blouses, and delicate fabrics. She chose a camisole, jeans, and a fancy blouse. As soon as we came home, she rushed to her room to put on the lacy camisole. Posing in front of the mirror she smiled. "I look pretty!"

Ten days later, Cody orchestrated one of the sweetest birthdays in my memory. I'd heard her whispering to Dennis several times the preceding week. I couldn't hear details, but I knew she was planning something for Friday, the night before my thirty-fifth birthday. Her friend Penny was staying overnight. Dennis and I went out with friends.

Returning from the movie, we found the living room and dining room decorated with crepe paper and Cody's drawings. A happy birthday sign hung over the archway between the rooms. Bowls of cookies and potato chips sat on the table. The house was quiet, with no sign of Cody.

Suddenly, her bedroom door flew open and out came Milka, Dan, and a parade of little kids wearing colorful costumes: Cody, Penny, Kari, Amy, Anna, Beth, Krissy, Katie, and Adam. Neighbor moms Robbie and Kate followed them.

Cody directed me to sit in a chair labeled "Birthday Girl." A sign on the wall had everyone's signature, including the dogs. Each child presented a gift. The first was a piece of bubblegum. I received a dishtowel, a piece of toffee, and cross-stitched balloons in a small frame. After presents, there was entertainment. The three youngest—Katie, Kris, and Adam—had painted faces and were dressed as clowns named Smiles, Winky, and Ping Ping. Their comedy skit involved honking each other's noses.

The oldest Newberg girls performed together. Amy and Beth twirled batons while Kari beat plastic bowls with spoons and chanted an original poem. Penny was draped in scarves and wore rosaries around her neck. Hers was fancy dancing, and little Katie joined her. Katie did a moonwalk and somersaults. She had a wild, sweet grin as she spun around and kept her eyes on me. I laughed hard and kept laughing as we ate cake.

Dennis's most important research project that year was with a university in Australia. When he'd been there before Christmas, he was asked to return again for several months if possible. Though our marriage was becoming stronger than ever, our counselor suggested we examine options other than spending months apart. We couldn't all go to Australia for so long. I'd lose my new job, and taking Cody there for an extended period was too complicated.

After much discussion, we found an acceptable compromise: I'd go with Dennis to Australia for five weeks in the early part of the summer while a trusted friend stayed with Cody and the dogs. Dennis would remain for another month after I came home. He'd be home by Cody's birthday at the end of the summer. All three of us would go to Australia for two weeks at Christmas.

Before leaving for Australia, I packed Cody's things for her twelve days at camp. I wrote a manual of instructions with medical information for our friend Reba, who was staying with Cody while I was gone. Little Dan was more anxious than usual and threw up several times as Dennis and I prepared to leave. Cody held him on her lap and assured him, "Mom and Dad will be back soon."

I called home from Australia when Cody returned from camp. She said, "I swam every day, and Robin was a counselor again, so I had fun." Cody had already called friends and written a two-page letter to Robin.

Everything sounded good whenever I called Cody, until the end of each conversation. She tended to throw in some horrible bit of news just before hanging up. At the end of the first call Cody said, "Bye, Mom. By the way, the plumber just left; it's okay now." Another call ended with, "See ya. I choked today at the restaurant, but I felt a lot better after I threw up."

Before the last leg of my flight home, I called from Los Angeles. Cody said, "I can't wait for you to be home! I want to know exactly when you'll be here. Ring the doorbell instead of using your key, so I'll know."

When the taxi dropped me off, Cody greeted me at the door. We hugged hello. As I kissed and hugged the dogs, she asked, "Can I offer you something to eat?"

I'd been gone only a few weeks, but my daughter appeared to have matured from twelve to twenty. In the next few days, she did things that I'd not seen before. She washed dishes, cleaned the sink, and made her bed. When friends came to dinner that weekend, Cody cleared the table and did other little extras. On the weekend, she hooked up the hose and, along with her friends, washed the car. She was drenched, exhausted but cheerful, and the car was clean. I commented, "You sure grew up while I was gone."

"It's no big deal, Mom. I'm almost a teenager." She put on her headset, closed her eyes, and sang along with The Jets.

Cody had described feeling panicky a few times before the end of the previous school year, so I'd scheduled an evaluation with a psychologist for later in the summer. I didn't want her to suffer the way I had with anxiety attacks.

After an interview and a battery of assessments, IQ tests, and other indicators, the psychologist reported "statistically significant discrepancies between Cody's verbal and performance IQs." The written summary concluded, "Standardized intelligence testing may not accurately reflect the intellectual potential for a child with spina bifida."

This was not new or useful information. We'd heard this sort of thing from the time Cody first started school. Standardized tests are not designed for the non-standard kid.

The psychologist didn't think Cody needed treatment or medication for anxiety. She suggested deep breathing. One helpful suggestion was that Cody might benefit from more female role models.

I called Big Brothers and Big Sisters. A match was found almost immediately. Cody was assigned a Big Sister to spend time with her on a regular basis as her mentor and friend.

JP was an attractive young flight attendant. When she came to our house for the first time, she directed her conversation to Cody. That was a refreshing sign. Anyone with a family member or friend with a disability knows how often others direct conversation to companions present instead of to the individual. Restaurant servers often ignored Cody and asked me, "What does she want?"

JP told Cody, "I've never had a friend in a wheelchair. I'm excited to be your friend."

Cody came to work with me on her thirteenth birthday. My coworkers had decorations, cake, and presents for her: a pink sweater and a backpack full of school supplies for the start of seventh grade. When we came home, Cody made an off-balance turn as she wheeled up the backyard sidewalk. She flipped backwards and her head slammed onto the cement.

I picked her up and rushed her inside. She was dizzy and nauseous. It was the worst blow to the head Cody ever had. We both worried that her shunt might have been affected. But the swollen bump that formed was in a different spot. The doctor said to watch her for two or three hours. After that, he was no longer concerned. The initial crashing pain took an hour to subside. Cody was left with a headache that threatened to dampen her birthday celebration. Five friends were supposed to spend the night.

I held an icepack on Cody's head. She still had a throbbing headache when the doorbell rang and a box of presents arrived from Tad, who was now working for Catholic Charities in Houston. Cody's girlfriends were due to start arriving, so I asked her if she thought we should cancel the party.

"No way! I'm finally a teenager. This is an important birthday."

The girls enjoyed pizza, cake, and goodies. I spread blankets and pillows on the living room floor and moved Cody's and Rachel's wheelchairs out of the way. All six girls stretched out to watch videos and eat Popsicles. After the second movie, I made a late night snack of melted cheese on nacho chips. I went to bed after the third movie. The girls giggled and talked into the night. Cody never mentioned her head bump again.

Dennis was only home a short time before he had to return to Australia that fall for further work. Between trips, we attended a parent-teacher conference at Cody's school. Anwatin was the designated junior high for mainstreamed students. Rachel and Cody's other friends from Dowling were now together again in the same school.

The teacher said Cody was doing well in seventh grade and readily helped others with their work. Rachel was in Cody's typing class. Typing was slow and difficult for Rachel, so Cody explained the keyboard to her and helped her during class.

The teacher added, "Although Cody is doing very well in all her classes, she never turns in her homework assignments."

Surprised, I said, "Cody always tells me she doesn't have homework."

The teacher explained that homework assignments were written on the board each day.

That night, I asked Cody, "Why do you always tell me you don't have homework?"

She said, "They don't give me any at this school."

I told her about the assignments on the board. Cody said, "Those are for the other kids, not me."

As we discussed it further, I learned that, in fifth and sixth grades, Cody had been given different homework than the non-disabled children. Although assignments for the rest of the class were put on the board, Cody's homework was explained to her individually. Often the work differed entirely. She naturally assumed this was still the case in junior high. Now understanding that assignments on the board were also meant for her, she turned in her homework every day.

Cody was prescribed a new wheelchair at her next outpatient clinic appointment. Her heavy Everest Jennings chair was replaced by a lightweight Quickie 2 sports model. Instead of gray metal, Cody had a color choice. She chose a blazing fluorescent pink to offset the black seat, pedals, and back. The chair was easier for Cody to maneuver, and easy for me to fold and lift into the trunk of our car. Whenever Cody outgrew a wheelchair, we kept it as a backup until the next time, when it was donated. The spare chair came in handy when a tire went flat or brakes were out of adjustment. Cody's lighter chair arrived in time for our Oz Christmas trip.

Colder-than-usual temperatures and bitter windchill during November and December increased the allure of an Australian summer. When we reached Los Angeles and boarded our nonstop flight to Sydney, there were plenty of empty seats. Dennis stretched across an entire row of middle seats and slept through most of the flight. Cody's Foley catheter and drainage bag worked well. She listened to music on her headset, read, or slept. I did the same. Cody laughed when I reminded her how she kept me awake talking until just before the plane landed on our trip to Australia when she was seven.

A neighbor boy had constructed a temporary wooden ramp to the back door of Dennis's mother's house for this visit. On our last trip, Cody felt insecure in Gwen's home. The dog had escaped from the yard while Dennis and I were away with friends. Cody cried frantically when everyone left the house to chase the dog.

She later said, "What if there was a fire, and no one was there to get me out?"

Cody, Dennis, and I often discussed plans to escape if there was a fire at school or at friends' homes. We made sure there was an adult to rescue Cody if she couldn't get out on her own. We had similar conversations on airplanes and in shopping malls. Unless a parent was with her, Cody avoided places she couldn't escape from without help.

On Christmas day we went to the beach. Cody saw her cousins almost every day; Melissa stayed the night with her on Gwen's veranda. Cody wore her earphones most of the time and rocked to the beat of whatever music blared in her headset.

A drive around the countryside ended up in Kuppacumbalong, a tiny town where we bought presents for friends at home who were staying with our dogs. Cody made purchases with her own money. She selected a sundress and a poster of a wallaroo. We saw horses and donkeys grazing in fields belonging to friends in Gosford. Cody played tambourines and flutes with the little girls who lived there. Dennis stopped the car at Towradgi Beach on the way to the airport because Cody wanted to see the ocean a last time and fill a container with sand. "I love to fly," she said when she was buckled up in her airplane seat, wearing her headset, sipping a Diet Coke.

Our trip home was without incident except when I emptied Cody's Foley bag. The plastic bag filled up quickly because she was drinking so much. I didn't hold up the bag high enough and a fountain of urine squirted all over my foot, Cody's, the floor, and whatever else was down there. Cody was terribly amused by my floundering around under the blanket as I tried to dry off everything.

In the baggage area at the Minneapolis/St. Paul airport, a small boy about three or four stared at Cody and pointed at her wheelchair. She smiled and said hello. He gazed at Cody as she told him, "I have this chair on wheels so I can go places even though my legs don't work."

As the boy stepped closer, his mother pulled him away.

This sort of interaction happened frequently in public places. Cody always focused on the children and took no offense.

Chapter 11

Typical?

CODY BECAME what I thought of as a typical teenager. She was particular about her appearance, wanted her ears pierced, and spent her allowance on earrings to match whatever she wore. She had occasional problems with girlfriends and kids at school. She got up early for the school bus, was tired a lot, felt bored and confused, obsessed about boys, and sometimes hated her parents.

As a consequence of not cleaning her room as I'd requested for several days, I didn't allow Cody to watch one of her favorite television shows. She left a note: "Dear Marly [She called me Marly when she was angry.], I'm going on a long walk and may never come back. If you think I'm teasing, you are sadly mistaken. If you love me, you will come and find me. Cody." She drew a happy face next to her name.

Another note, when she was fourteen, read: "I'm sick and tired of you ordering me around. I'm not going to take it anymore. You will never find me, because I am going far. I need some fun and I'm going to have it whether you like it or not. P.S. Tell Dennis bye for me."

I usually found her halfway up the block and talked her into coming home.

Cody went to and from school on different buses than other kids rode. Her smaller buses were equipped with wheelchair lifts. The driver strapped down wheelchairs for safety while the bus was in motion. Cody and Donna, a girl in a motorized wheelchair, waited together for a bus home from school.

Although Cody had known Donna for years, they weren't close friends. But while talking one afternoon, Donna confided that the bus driver fondled her breasts when she was the only one on the bus. Due to her disability, she couldn't push the man's hands away. She was afraid to say anything to make him stop. Cody said, "That's horrible! You need to tell on that guy!"

Donna said, "I can't. He'll get mad; he could hurt me."

Cody spun her chair around and said, "Come with me."

"No, wait!" Donna was alarmed, but she followed Cody to the principal's office.

Cody told the principal what was happening to Donna, and the driver was fired the same day. Cody arrived home later than usual that afternoon.

She angrily told me, "I can't believe the nerve of that creep. He scared Donna so much she didn't know what to do."

"I'm really proud of you, babe. You did a good thing."

Cody steamed, "I'd like to punch that creep."

Mom stayed at our house for a couple of days that spring while my father had some business in southern Minnesota. We enjoyed some girls-only chats. Cody took Mom to see her school one morning, but the fun was cut short when Cody developed a bad headache. Within two hours it was obvious from her sunsetting eyes and grogginess that her shunt wasn't working. Mom had never before been with Cody during a medical emergency.

At the hospital, my mother was quiet as she followed Cody's gurney up and down the hallways and watched the tests and procedures. Her face was taut as I explained the reasons for what we were doing at each step.

Cody lay still with her eyes shut and was hard to rouse by the time she was taken into surgery at 3:15 in the afternoon. Mom sat with me in the family room while I did homework. I had started graduate school that year. I found it easier to focus on a class paper than to think about what was happening to Cody.

The doctor came out at 3:50. Thirty-five minutes from start to finish was the fastest brain surgery Cody ever had. The neurosurgeon said he found blood in the shunt, that Cody must have had a recent fall or blow to the head. I remembered the fall on her thirteenth birthday, but that was eighteen months ago. When I asked Cody, though, she remembered bumping her head at school two days before.

As Cody rested in her hospital bed, Mom turned to look at me and said, "That was hard." It was her only comment, and she was sincere.

By the time Dad returned from southern Minnesota the next night, Cody was home and we all went to a movie. That weekend, Cody attended a Jets concert as part of the Girl Scouts 75th anniversary celebration. In a few short days, we went from happy times to scary emergency, and back to happy times. Just like that.

When I told my teacher about Cody's emergency surgery, Marcia said, "I can't even imagine how difficult it must be to have your child's life threatened over and over the way Cody's has been. It must be frightening for you."

I didn't know how to respond when people said things like that to me.

She added, "It must be frightening for Cody also, since she realizes the dangers, too."

Marcia's comment made me wonder how much Cody thought about things like that. The following night I was in bed with a cold and stomachache. Cody was in her bed and we talked back and forth across the hall. I said, "I love you, babe. I am sure glad you're okay. I was really scared when you had to have surgery."

Cody answered, "I wasn't really scared this time. I knew I'd get through it. After all, I've been on death row before."

Our family took part in a study of teenagers with spina bifida. We were asked to complete a follow-up survey. I was in bed, still feeling queasy, when Cody came in to chat. Our floors weren't carpeted, so she scooted easily in a seated position from her room. She brought the forms with her. She said she was bored and didn't want to finish the survey. I offered to help and she handed me the papers. Cody rested her head on the bed and looked serious as she idly scratched Milka behind the ears while we finished the questionnaire. I asked, "Did something about these questions bother you?"

She nodded. "I don't like thinking about being disabled."

But she agreed to finish in case it would help other kids. We chatted until after ten that night. Cody said she wanted to take singing lessons. I liked her idea; she'd have fun and develop lung capacity. I called the next day to arrange them, and drove her downtown to an arts center every Tuesday evening for her singing lessons. Cody's goal was to sing "Silent Night" for Tad's family at Christmas.

On her days off from school, Cody came to work with me. There she met Elizabeth, a coworker who hosted a weekly program called *Saturday's Child* on a listener-supported radio station. She invited Cody to bring some music selections to play on the air the following week.

"Sure!" Cody said, "That would be fun."

She chose several of her favorites: Lionel Ritchie's "Hello," "Let's Hear It for the Boy" from the movie *Footloose*, Climax's "I Miss You," and "Glory of Love" by Peter Cetera. On the air, Cody introduced each song and identified the singer. Amy Newberg came along, too, and read poems. At the end of the show, Cody was asked to come back every week as a regular co-host. Amy or Kari Newberg joined her for several programs, playing music or discussing relevant topics, like tornados. I tape-recorded the programs and noticed over time that Cody sounded more and more professional as she said things like, "The time is ten-fifteen. You are listening to *Saturday's Child*. This is Cody."

At the end of eighth grade, Cody won an award for "outstanding" work in Industrial Technology. She was invited to an award presentation with members of the school board in attendance. A NASA astronaut, Colonel Loren J. Shriver, spoke at the ceremony and showed a film about outer space. Cody's friend Lewis and his mother sat with us.

Cody and Lewis played adaptive sports together in junior high. He was a handsome boy with huge brown eyes and long lashes. He tilted his chin down and looked up with a broad smile with the same shy charm as Princess Diana. Lewis had a disability that impaired his bone growth. To walk, he turned his body at the hips to swing each leg forward.

He and Cody planned to go to the same camp that summer. When Lewis had neck surgery, Cody visited him at Shriners Hospital. We'd become friends with Lewis's mother, Cynthia, who joked around with Cody like a girlfriend.

When her name was called at the ceremony, Cody wheeled forward, accepted her certificate and shook hands with the astronaut. The following week, she visited NASA.

Tad had been trying for months to arrange for Cody to visit him in Houston. But I wasn't comfortable sending her on a plane by herself. Cody suggested bringing Amy. Though she was a couple of years younger than Cody, Amy was responsible and mature for her age. She knew Cody could have medical emergencies and had sometimes visited her in the hospital.

I tried to anticipate every possible travel barrier and safety threat. Tad researched and identified a hospital and neurosurgeon in Houston in case of a shunt problem. We created a contingency plan if the plane was diverted to another city for any reason, and Cody promised to call me when her plane landed in Texas.

Dennis was at a conference in Russia so I took the girls to the airport. I was allowed onto the plane to help Cody settle in her seat. I showed the flight attendant how Cody could transfer in and out of an airplane seat, and demonstrated how to fold and stow the wheelchair.

Cody made sure she was cathed right before the flight and again as soon as she landed. She wore an incontinent brief with extra padding in case of a delay. Tad met the plane in Houston and went onboard to bring Cody off the plane in her wheelchair.

Thankfully, there were no mishaps. Cody returned home wearing a baseball cap with a NASA insignia. Her now light-auburn hair had blonde highlights from the sunshine. Her skin was a golden tan. The girls had a great vacation and told funny stories about adventures with Tad. They had sung together at a recording booth in Houston. Cody convinced Tad to let the girls curl his hair and put makeup on his face. She had pictures to prove it. Cody and Amy talked about NASA on the radio show that week and played a tape of Tad singing Lionel Ritchie's "All Night Long."

Cody made more recordings at a singing booth at the Minnesota State Fair later in the summer. Since her birthday fell in the last week of

August, the fair was a regular part of her celebration. Prior to the year Cody turned fifteen, the singing booth was up a step, making wheelchair entry impossible. She had written a letter and made several calls about it. That year Cody was able to wheel into the booth. She, Amy, and Kari sang duets and trios and played some of the tapes on the radio show.

At her first singing lesson the previous spring, Cody wasn't able to sing more than a few words without taking a breath. But after months of daily voice exercises and rehearsing, she could now sing entire phrases in one breath.

Cody started ninth grade at South High, the magnet school for talented kids and the designated high school for students with disabilities. The transition to high school was a bigger deal for me than it was for Cody. Some of the older boys were huge, with facial hair.

She liked being one of the big kids, and Lewis was in some of her classes. She had a bigger crush on him after being together with him at summer camp. Cody had crushes on other boys, too. Many of the objects of her affection were not aware of her interest, but I heard about them almost every day after school.

Early in her freshman year, Cody told me two "mean boys" picked on her each day in the hall. She refused to tell me the nasty names the boys called her, but she said, "They stand on either side of me, crowd into me, and give me a hard time."

I suggested she tell a teacher, but Cody thought that was advice for a kid.

One day as the boys taunted her, she said in a strong voice, "You better get away from me, or you'll be sorry."

They jeered and one boy said, "Oh, right. Like you could hurt anybody!"

Cody smiled as she told me, "I decided to let them have it."

Cody's undeniably strong arms were at the boys' groin level. She elbowed both boys at the same time. She laughed describing the way the boys yowled.

"You should have seen their faces, Mom. I don't think they'll bother me again."

During an October parent-teacher meeting, Dennis and I were shown the results of Cody's wide-range interest tests. Her top interests were identified as child psychology, office work, and horticulture. The first two made sense to me. Cody loved small children and anticipated their needs and interests. She enjoyed using the computer in my office at work. She offered to stuff envelopes and file papers for me. Horticulture seemed the odd choice. Any plant in her room died from neglect. We chatted while I weeded the garden but she never wanted her hands in the dirt. These tests didn't show what I thought was obvious—Cody cared most about *music*. In her journal she wrote that listening to music was her favorite thing to do.

She was three when I first found her crying as she listened to a record. I asked what was wrong. She couldn't speak, but she cried harder during the song's refrain. I had asked if the music made her cry. Her lower lip jutted out as she nodded. I hugged Cody and said, "Aww, honey, it's a touching song, isn't it?" At times a repeated phrase evoked her emotional response, something in a ballad, love song, or nursery rhyme. Other times, instead of lyrics, chord changes or sweet-sounding instrumentation triggered her weeping with the music.

In Philadelphia at Christmas, the Cornell family cheered Cody's performance of "Silent Night." We stayed with the family of her former babysitters. Cody thought the boys were cute when she was seven; now all three were handsome young men. Middle brother, Pierce, played guitar and sang for Cody. On the flight home, she talked about his music and decided he was the cutest.

Before the plane landed, Cody's head was throbbing in pain. By the time we were home in Minneapolis, she couldn't raise her eyes at all. We rushed her to St. Paul Children's Hospital.

Chapter 12

Days and Nights

DENNIS AND I KNEW how critical it was for Cody to have brain surgery within a few hours of the first symptoms that her shunt wasn't working. At fifteen, Cody now had a clearer understanding of her vulnerability, as well. We were more than familiar with the dozens of questions asked by residents, medical students, nurses, and others who came and went through the evening. To save repeating myself, I gave the doctor in charge our typed summary of Cody's medical issues, surgeries, hospitalization dates, allergies and immunizations. Otherwise, it was hard to remember all details that might be important in any given situation. Doctors routinely commented that the summary was invaluable and often suggested useful additions. One surgeon recommended noting that Cody had had blood transfusions in the past. Another said I should highlight her allergies in larger letters. I kept the summary on a single page, had multiple copies on hand, and provided updated versions to her caregivers.

The neurosurgeon decided against shunt-revision surgery that night. He saw no obvious obstruction or mechanical malfunction in the shunt. Multiple images on the CAT scan film showed two enlarged black areas, the ventricles, where cerebrospinal fluid had accumulated in her brain. The shunt apparatus appeared like a bent drinking straw poking into one of the ventricles. Cody had no fever or other indication of infection. Despite her painful headache and inability to look up, she remained lucid and con-scious. The doctor suggested that the lack of progression in her symptoms could mean the problem might correct itself; perhaps a small obstruction had flushed through the shunt. He placed Cody under observation.

Before he left, I asked the doctor every question I could think of. I asked if airplane travel could have triggered an increase in intracranial pressure. The doctor didn't think there was a connection, but I continued to wonder about that. For now, all I could do was wait—not my best skill when my daughter was hurting.

Dennis went home and I stayed overnight with Cody. As with each of her sixteen previous hospitalizations, we alternated spending the nights with her.

A nurse came into the darkened room every two hours to shine a flashlight in Cody's eyes, checking for signs of neurological change, further increase in intracranial pressure, or loss of consciousness. Cody and I held hands in the dark. We spoke in soft voices off and on through the night.

The "parent's" cot between Cody's bed and the window was on a distinct slant. If I relaxed, I rolled back toward the window. I felt cold air leaking in. The temperature outside was dropping. I tried to resist the cot's slant in search of a comfortable position. I exaggerated my predicament to entertain Cody. I pretended to fall back toward the windowsill and then pull myself toward her bedrail, reaching like a rope-climber, gasping and panting as if it required monumental effort. Always a sucker for slapstick, she laughed in spite of her pain.

I tucked the bedspread behind my back to keep from rolling toward the window. I asked Cody, "Remember when you made me drive by Orlando's house?"

Cody thought Orlando was cute. She had wanted to see where he lived. As I'd driven up his street and found his address, she asked me to drive around the block a few times then through the back alley. As we approached Orlando's alley garage on the right, Cody said, "Stop! Someone's in the backyard!" I braked and Cody threw herself down on the seat, leaving me looking straight at the person in the yard. I scowled, "Cody!" She dissolved in laughter.

I now teased, "That person probably thought I was a stalker!"

Cody smiled again, but kept her eyes shut.

By morning, she was no better or worse. The neurosurgeon decided to operate but he found nothing wrong with the shunt. He reinserted the apparatus into her head and closed the incision. He suggested that perhaps the problem was gone and the worst of it was that the right side of Cody's head was shaved. That was bad enough for a fifteen-year-old.

Her headache was relieved slightly after surgery, but within hours the pain was just as severe as the night before. When Cody tried to look up, her eyes darted instead to the side. She lay still with her eyes closed. The blinds were shut and the lights were off in her room. For the rest of the day she winced whenever her IV pump beeped.

That evening, Dennis and I sat on either side of her bed in the dark, each holding one of Cody's hands, encouraging her to sleep. When the neurosurgeon finally called in for a progress report, I spoke to him on the phone at the nurses' station across the hall from Cody's room.

"What should we watch for? What might happen?"

He said, "I don't know. Wait to see what happens. We'll handle it when the time comes."

No matter how I rephrased my questions, he yielded no information about what to expect or what he was thinking. I reminded myself that we chose this doctor in the first place because of his stellar reputation, not his personality. I had no choice but to trust his expertise and pray for him to do the right thing to help Cody. I was glad the light was dim so Cody couldn't see that I was crying when I returned to her room. I leaned close to her face and whispered, "I know this is tough, sweetie. You're being terrific. You're always terrific. I love you."

Cody answered in a sleepy voice, "I don't know what's going to happen to me."

I felt the familiar ache I'd known often in our fifteen years together. I thought of it as mother-ache, but fathers felt it, too. I wanted to save my child, protect her from this hurt and fear. I wished I could trade places with her. I hesitated to leave, even though it was Dennis's turn to stand guard on the parent's cot for the night. I prayed, "Please, God, take care of my girl."

Cody said, "Kiss the dogs for me."

Sometime after ten, I drove home. A nurse checked Cody's vital signs every two hours. She and Dennis slept.

Our poor dogs were crazy with excitement and anxious for attention. Milka and Dan had been alone for hours and hours in the past two days. I was thankful that our neighbors, Art and Robbie, offered to let them out in the afternoons. The dogs had stayed with friends during our ten-day trip back east, and they weren't yet accustomed to being home.

Home didn't feel normal to me either. I fed the dogs and listened to phone messages left on the answering machine. I appreciated that machine. A few friends and relatives left good wishes and asked how Cody was doing. I went to bed at midnight with a dog under each arm, praying that in the morning I'd hear Cody was fine.

Each time Cody was in the hospital, nurses gave me forms to fill out that included a section to list patient's siblings. I usually filled in our dogs' names. Though meant in fun, it was also true. Cody and I both liked to hold a dog in our arms at bedtime. As I held Milka and Dan close that night, I drifted off, picturing angels surrounding Cody's hospital bed.

At 2:00 a.m., a nurse took Cody's vitals and left the room. Only a moment later, Dennis looked at Cody's silhouette against the light from the corridor. He thought at first he was silly to stare so intently, but he couldn't see her covers moving. He jumped up and looked closer. Even in the darkened room he saw that Cody had stopped breathing. Dennis screamed for help.

Clinicians swarmed around Cody. She was "stabilized" at the same moment that Dennis reached me by phone. He spoke calmly, but I was shaking so much I could hardly stand. Within moments I was in the bathroom, my body wracked by a spontaneous purge.

Outside, the temperature was 30 below with a wind-chill of 50 below, the coldest night in years. Travel advisories warned it was dangerous to go out. Dennis didn't want me to drive to the hospital. He reminded me that I'd been up all night the night before, and I should try to sleep. He said Cody was fine now, being watched closely. There was nothing I could do, or even any room for me now that she'd been moved to the pediatric intensive care unit (PICU). He sounded decisive and strong; I agreed to stay home. He promised to call with any further news.

After hanging up, I moved in slow motion. The dogs sat together, watching me weave through the house as I tried to figure out what I should do. I wanted to be ready to go if Dennis called again. I pulled on tights, knee socks and jeans, a T-shirt and sweater. With two layers of clothes, I climbed back into bed. I lay under the covers praying and crying until 3:00 a.m. when I thought to call Tad in Houston. He'd just seen Cody at his family gathering at Christmas. I knew that, despite the late hour, he'd want to know what happened. I couldn't stop crying as I told him. Tad said, "Oh no!" and began to cry.

I promised to call him when there was any change in Cody's condition. I hung up and pulled the covers over me. Rocking and hugging Milka and Dan, I tried to sleep.

I phoned the hospital at six in the morning. Cody was still "stable." I called my brother in St. Louis. Charlie was now connected to larger communities of Christians who prayed for people in trouble. I wanted all the forces for good in the universe to be focused on saving my girl. I imagined dozens of people I'd never met, an army of faithful people, praying for Cody.

Charlie said a prayer right then on the phone and assured me that God was taking care of everything. He pointed out the miracle that Dennis awoke at the exact moment to save Cody's life. Angel shivers moved through my body as I realized it was true. *Dennis had saved her life.*

I began to feel hopeful. I reminded myself that Cody's life had been a string of miracles from the beginning. I again envisioned angels posted around her like soldiers prepared for battle to protect her. I called Father Dan at church. He was surprised to hear how serious things had become. The second I hung up, the phone rang. This time Dennis was crying. Cody had stopped breathing again. I cried, "No!"

"They're still trying to stabilize her . . . you'd better come."

Before hanging up we quickly said a few things to reassure each other. I called our neighbor Art to ask for a ride to the hospital, and ran out the back door.

Art's eyes mirrored my fear as we sped to St. Paul. But in the middle of the Lake Street Bridge over the Mississippi River, the car stopped dead in the freezing cold. At a standstill on an empty bridge, we were suspended between cement-colored sky and a frozen river. Snowflakes cut through the gray morning air. I felt an odd calm. I couldn't control a broken-down car or the weather. Art jumped out, opened my door and yelled, "We'd better start hoofing it."

I climbed out into the icy air and said, "Wait, Art. Where can we run? We'd better hail down a car for a ride back to my car."

Our Toyota was in the garage at home. I wondered why it hadn't occurred to me to take it in the first place. Tears were freezing on my face.

Art ran out in front of the first oncoming vehicle. He waved his arms and blocked the car from swerving around him on the bridge. Art was a big guy. He must have looked like a wild man to the two wide-eyed young women whose car skidded to a stop in front of him. His eyes conveyed the urgency of our predicament. He blurted out our need, and we were driven back to the house. In silent sympathy, one of the women reached to me in the backseat and held my hand as we drove. She asked my daughter's name.

Once in the Toyota, Art pressed hard on the gas pedal and we roared toward the hospital. Driving so fast on frozen streets, I imagined us crashing, and poor Dennis losing his daughter and wife in one day. I told Art to relax and drive the way he normally does.

"This *IS* how I normally drive!"

I felt a pang of guilt for putting Art in this position. I knew he felt terrible; he shared my fear for Cody. Art was a gentle, strong man with five girls of his own. I thought how lucky we were to have such dear friends close by.

Art dropped me at the hospital entrance. I ran inside and asked the first person I saw in scrubs how to find the PICU. As I rushed toward the unit, I searched nurses' faces to see if I could read that someone had just died.

A room on the far side of the PICU was full of people. I saw Dennis's wonderful relieved face. Cody had been stabilized only a moment before. She was now on a respirator, hooked up to monitors, another IV, and some machines I didn't recognize.

I took Cody's hand and kissed her cheek. She gripped my hand. Her eyes conveyed fear and surprise. Our faces were touching, and I kissed her again. I kept my lips close to her cheek and told her that she had stopped breathing, but that she was fine now.

She gestured with her hand toward the respirator. I could see she hated the plastic tubing that invaded her throat. I told her it was helping her breathe. Monitors on either side of the bed made clicking noises. Wavy fluorescent green lines formed patterns that moved across the screen. Even though the room was full of people in scrubs and white coats, the only other sound was a machine making gurgling noises.

The emergency care physician and a neurologist took turns telling me what had happened and shared their amazement that Cody had stopped breathing. She'd been alert and conscious only moments before. Someone said it made no sense.

Convinced finally that the near-death event was done, the caregivers around Cody's bed shuffled out of the room one by one. Their storm of activity had saved her. She was about to go into surgery; her neurosurgeon was on the way. The doctor in charge said he wanted to put in an arterial IV. He told Dennis and me to leave the room.

Cody tightened her grip on my hand. I said I'd stay, as I'd always done during procedures in preparation for surgery. I didn't want to leave her alone when she was scared. I insisted on staying no matter how gross the procedure. It wasn't that I had a strong stomach or was desensitized to blood and gore. It was more about being able to focus on Cody's face, look into her eyes, and blur out the rest. With everything invasive that I'd watched doctors do to Cody, I held my facial expression in calmness because Cody was looking at me. If I did not appear alarmed, hopefully she would not be alarmed. If I held onto her, and behaved as if all was well, then all would be well. It seemed to work. But this time Cody had almost died. A machine was breathing for her. Everyone's nerves were on high alert. The doctor insisted a third time saying, "We lose more parents than kids doing this procedure."

We'd heard that old saw before, but this time it wasn't worth arguing. Cody and I exchanged an accepting glance. A nurse pulled the curtain shut, blocking my view.

Dennis and I used those moments to find Art, tell him that Cody was all right and thank him. He had parked our car in the hospital lot. He gave us the keys and left to take a cab home.

Cody was taken into surgery within the hour and given a new shunt, this time on the left side of her head. Having the rest of her head shaved became the most minor of our concerns.

After surgery, the anesthetic wore off quickly. Cody was taken back to the PICU. Her headache was almost gone. Dennis and I were told that Cody would be on the respirator for at least two days, until doctors were sure she could breathe on her own.

The intracranial pressure, which had stopped Cody's breathing, had also pressed hard on her optic nerve. She could not see anything in front of her. If she tilted her head from side to side, using peripheral vision, she could make out the large letters on an alphabet I drew on a sketchpad. Cody lifted her right arm with its plastic tubing attachments and pointed to the letters one by one. She took several minutes to spell out "I am scared" and "I am afraid I will die."

Dennis and I leaned close and assured her she was alive and well. I told Cody what a miracle it was that Dennis woke up and looked at her just as she stopped breathing.

The emergency care physician later told Dennis that Cody would have died if he had not noticed the first time she stopped breathing. The nurse that night wasn't due to return for two more hours to recheck Cody's vital signs. The doctor added, "People think hospitals are the safest places, but it's not true. There are so many people to care for; so much can happen."

I appreciated his honesty and his candor. He was one of the doctors I could trust. I made a mental note to send a thank-you letter to the hospital and mention the names of this physician and the others who assisted in saving Cody's life that morning.

Cody remained attached to the various machines, two IVs, a nose tube and the puffing blue respirator, for two more days. She was frustrated and uncomfortable the entire time. Her nurse told me how unusual it was for a patient to be awake on a respirator. "People on respirators are usually unconscious and unaware of their discomfort."

Cody was *acutely* aware of her discomfort, and she used her time to make sure that I knew it, too. She painstakingly spelled out, "Get me out of here" several times, and "I mean it."

I told her how sorry I was that she was so miserable. I hoped that the more irritable she was, the more likely her condition was improving. That was often the case in the past.

There was no parent's cot, slanted or otherwise, in the PICU—only a chair. I stayed by Cody's side each day, read to her, told her how the dogs were doing and what friends had called.

When the machines were disconnected and Cody could finally speak, she said the respirator had scared her the most. She was afraid she'd swallow it and die. She'd seen a character on *General Hospital* on a respirator, and he had died.

Now she was freed. My relief was immense. A feeling of reverie and gratefulness spread over everything. I'd felt that way before over the years. As I pushed through the hospital entrance with cards and goodies for Cody, I felt connected to each person I saw. A painless ache followed me down hospital hallways. I wondered what the woman with the knitting needles was making and who the man in the gift shop was visiting. I saw the tightness in the shoulders of a doctor in green scrubs who leaned against a wall. I whispered a quick prayer for him. I imagined a family for the gray-haired lady who limped as she pushed a tall metal cart. A smile exchanged with a woman on the elevator felt more like an embrace. Snowflakes sparkled outside, but the bitter cold didn't touch me during those days and nights right after Cody didn't die.

A recreational therapist called the "Play Lady" visited and asked if there was anything Cody could think of that would make her feel better. Cody said, "I just want to see my dogs."

Play Lady left for a few minutes and came back with news. Dennis and I could bring Milka and Dan to the unit later that day. Cody's face lit up for the first time since the serious ordeal began. When the dogs arrived, Milka and Dan lay on the bed and Cody immediately fell asleep.

A nurse gave me a message that someone called to ask about Cody. She was one of the young women who picked up Art and me from the bridge the morning Cody stopped breathing. I called back to thank her again for the ride. She had prayed and worried about us. She said her small taste of our experience had changed her life forever. *Mine, too.*

Chapter 13

Eyes and Hockey

CODY HELD HER HAND in front of her face and said, "All I can see is a giant black space blobs in my eyes. I can't see anything right in front of me."

She was about to be discharged from the hospital as soon as the neurosurgeon came to see her. Her doctor was always in a hurry. Dennis and I intended to make sure he answered *all* our questions this time; we wanted to understand what happened.

"I'm afraid I might stop breathing again. Make sure to ask about that."

When the physician arrived, he remained standing as I asked the first question on our list. "Has what happened to Cody's eyes occurred before in your experience?"

The doctor said, "Yes, but it's not common."

"What has been the typical resolution of these vision problems? What's the prognosis for Cody to regain normal sight?"

He said, "I don't remember. Almost anything can happen with shunts. I would defer to an ophthalmologist on that."

"Do you have any further thoughts on why Cody stopped breathing, and why she experienced vision complications?"

"Not really. Nothing about it makes sense." The doctor scratched his forehead. "What happened was very unusual. I'm not pleased with it."

"Are you aware of similar problems that could cause Cody to have other temporary or permanent disabilities?"

The doctor took a pen from his coat pocket, turned over a hospital menu, and sketched a profile of a human head. He explained that Cody's brain had an Arnold Chiari malformation commonly associated with spina bifida. "The position and shape of her brain is a factor in a buildup of cerebrospinal fluid." He indicated the spot in the back of the head where the lower part of the brain presses near the top of the spinal column. He pointed with the tip of his pen and said, "Too much pressure on that part of the brain can affect involuntary functions like respiration and vision."

This explanation further sharpened my sense of urgency about the associated dangers of future shunt breakdowns. I wasn't sure if Cody understood the implications or gravity of what she had just heard, but she knew enough to propose our next step. She said in a firm voice, "I want to talk to an eye doctor."

The neurosurgeon gave us the number of the "best" ophthalmologist in the Twin Cities. The first available appointment was early the next week.

Cody tired easily once she was home. That didn't seem unusual after two brain surgeries and several days on a respirator. Other than that, she was her cheery self. We shopped for hats and scarves to cover the shaved area on her head. She was worried about homework piling up, and she missed her school friends. Her teachers sent makeup assignments with a friend who rode Cody's bus.

The English teacher expected Cody to write daily in a journal. Mr. Debe said it was okay for her to dictate entries to me since she couldn't see. She wasn't sure how to begin, so I told her to say anything that came into her head. I wrote fast to keep up with her thoughts. She talked about animals, friends, boys. About her hospital experience, Cody said, "A couple of days ago, I had a power outage of my strength."

Her narrative strayed from the assigned topic to the image of a train traveling through wallpaper designs, from her white bedroom walls to her furniture, and on to our holiday vacation. "I wished I could have taken my bedroom out of my suitcase, so I could be by myself where no one could find me. I've realized that I'm one of those people who like to be by myself with no one to nag or bug me. I like to listen to music when I am stressed, crabby, or upset. When I grow up I'll probably be a radio announcer, singer, or child psychologist. I like little kids." She stopped. "I don't think I'm doing the assignment right. I'm only saying what I'm thinking."

"Keep going; you're doing great."

For her second assignment, she stayed on the topic of a poem, talking faster and faster. She paused and said, "My brain is still on the train."

After a full examination the following week, the ophthalmologist announced, "Cody has severe retinal hemorrhaging. Any improvement in her vision is unlikely for at least six months. I am sorry to tell you, but it's possible that her vision loss is permanent. She is legally blind."

Dennis and I exchanged a look of shock and horror. *Cody has been through enough—adding permanent blindness is too much!*

But before we could speak, Cody said, "There are cassettes at my school to help with homework. Maybe I can have classes with Orlando. He's legally blind. He gets books on tape."

Dennis and I looked at each other again. Who were we to be horrified? Cody's authentic response was positive and practical. I was moved to take her view as she accepted what came her way and pressed on with life.

That evening as we said bedtime prayers, I decided it was time again to pray for a miracle. I kissed Cody goodnight and called my brother Charlie. I asked him to please pray with his group for her eyesight. I called Mom, too. She was connected to several prayer chains. She said she'd activate our request and also pray with her Bible study group. Father Dan was already praying for Cody, and he requested parishioner prayers on her behalf that Sunday.

Cody was sometimes emotionally sensitive after major surgery. But this time she grew melancholy. I had to wake her more than once to get her moving in the mornings. For two weeks she called me every day at lunchtime from school—just to say hello, she said.

While Dennis was away for nine days on a business trip, Cody and I sat back on her bed or mine each evening and tried to figure out the source of her daily sadness. We examined all aspects of her scary hospital experience, but she didn't think that was it. I asked, "Is there a certain time of the day when you feel the saddest?"

"I feel bad at school."

"Tell me more about what happens at school."

As Cody described her school day, it dawned on me. Normal interactions with her friends between classes had changed now that she couldn't see. She couldn't see facial expressions and didn't know if others were looking at her when passing in the halls.

I'd focused on obvious physical and logistical problems with blindness, like how to get homework done, and what extra vitamins she could take for her eyes. I hadn't considered her potential social isolation. Cody was lonely! As the thought hit me, I explained my theory and put my arms around her. "No wonder you've been sad! I'm sorry you've been lonely, sweetie." She immediately released her upset in a flood of tears. Then we talked about what to do. I said I'd call in the morning to talk with the school counselor. Cody agreed to tell at least one friend the next day. She exhaled a deep breath as she laid her face on her pillow.

I heard the tub running at 6:00 a.m. Cody was up and ready for her morning routine. While I packed her lunch, she said, "I'm glad we figured out the problem."

I covered her cheeks with kisses that she accepted more readily than usual.

The school counselor talked to Cody's teachers that day, and the gym teacher had a word to the entire class. When she came home from school, Cody was smiling. "Lewis wants me to watch him play hockey at Thursday's game. Can you bring me home if I go?"

"Sure. Dennis will be home by then, so we can come, too, if you want."

"Cool!" Cody put the *Dirty Dancing* soundtrack in her boom box, moved her shoulders to the music, and began singing *"Let's hear it for the boy . . ."*

Even though she was unable to see in front of her, Cody was happy that Lewis wanted her to watch him play hockey. Lewis hung around mostly with Orlando at school. In addition to vision impairment, Orlando walked with crutches. He was shorter in stature due to whatever his disability was. Like Lewis, his upper body was muscular and strong. Cody had an intermittent flirtation and continuing friendship with both boys.

After school that Thursday, Dennis and I watched the adaptive floor hockey game from the middle of the first row of bleachers in the high school gym. Cody sat in front of us with two other girls near the score-keeper. She cheered and screamed for her team. She wheeled along the sidelines and moved her head back and forth, using peripheral vision to track the action. She provided us with tidbits of information about each of the members of our team between yells of encouragement to the players. She shouted, "Go for it!" and "You can do it!"

To play on the adaptive floor hockey team in high school, each player had to have a disability. Sometimes, the disability was not obvious to a spectator. I couldn't detect any physical impairment in either of the other team's best players. Cody confirmed that kids on visiting teams usually looked more able-bodied than those on her team. Both teams had players in wheelchairs to defend the goals. Goalie had been Cody's strongest position in gym class.

A Southeast Asian player ran by who appeared able-bodied. Cody said, "That's Long; he doesn't speak English."

Long flew around the gym like a one-man team, racing back and forth, grabbing the puck from anyone, even his own team members. His temper flew, too, as he banged his stick. It turned out he did speak a little English. He could be clearly heard shouting "shit" or "asshole" as he sped by. Sometimes he threw his hockey stick in a flourish of anger.

Dramatic temper displays were a specialty of the home team. Even Lewis threw his helmet and stick occasionally. He fell on his knees at one point in the action and rolled on the floor to emphasize his pain. I'd seen Dennis do that when he played soccer on a team in Bryn Mawr. He'd clutched his shin and crashed to the ground, punching the dirt—"all part of the drama of the sport," he told me later.

"Poor Lewis! Is he okay?" Cody turned her head from side to side to try to see him.

Back in action, Lewis ran by and said, "I'm okay, Cody."

Our team's goalie moved quickly in front of the net. When the puck whizzed past him to score a goal, he growled and spun his chair around, shaking his head with exaggerated shrugs.

Gary played forward center. He didn't become riled in any situation. His dad and brother came to most games and sat near us on the bleachers. Unlike Long, Gary never broke the running rule. When the puck came to Gary, he was steady and deliberate. He swung his stick and walked after the moving puck with heavy steps. Whether he hit or missed, nothing changed his expression, action, or speed.

Tuan scored the team's first goal. Cody said, "Tuan and Lewis are our best players."

Dennis pointed out to me how Lewis worked with Tuan to set up shots. Tuan made most of the goals our team scored. He had a withered hand and walked on one side of his right foot. My ankle hurt watching him hobble and pound down again and again on his bent foot.

Our team didn't have enough players to have substitutes. They all looked frayed and dog-tired as the game wore on. Between periods, Tuan lay back on the bleachers near Cody, puffing and sweating and clutching his side. But when the whistle blew, he resumed playing with enthusiasm. The boys stole quick glances at Cody and the two other girls.

Cody yelled, "Good job. Keep it up!"

The final score was 9–3. Our team lost despite the gallantry and theatrics. The athletes lined up and walked or wheeled past each other to shake hands. Our goalie had limited arm mobility. He thrust out his arm like a punch to shake hands—an apt visual expression of our team's frustration. Every time the team lost, the players felt so bad. Cody and the other girls were the first to rush out and say, "Great job!"

She wanted to join the team as soon as she could.

The doctor gasped when he reexamined Cody's eyes three weeks after her first ophthalmology appointment. She no longer strained or moved her head from side to side to see. After looking again into each eye, he turned and said, "She's gone from legally blind to normal vision in three weeks."

He said the massive floating hemorrhages in Cody's eyes were almost gone. Dennis, Cody, and I smiled wide at this miracle as the physician voiced his amazement. "The damage was so extensive!" He said it more than once.

I told him, "Hundreds of people have been praying for Cody's eyes."

The doctor looked at me and said, "Whoever was praying for her did a good job. They should keep it up. I have never seen anything like it."

Two days later Cody played her first hockey game as a goalie for the team. She blocked the net by wheeling back and forth, holding a hockey stick in her right hand. Several times, the puck banged her wheel and snapped away from the goal.

Cody focused on the action, yelled encouragement to her teammates, and cheered when someone scored. This was the first team sport Cody played that ended in a win. She shrieked with happiness and later called everyone she could think of to share news of the victory.

Chapter 14

Synchronized Miracles

FOR THE NEXT TWO WEEKS Dennis worked late at night in his study, so Cody and I had longer bedtime chats. At times I had trouble staying awake when she came to my room to talk about boys or whatever else was on her mind. We'd sometimes talk in her room. Her mood shifted once in a while, and she'd want me to leave. She flipped back and forth from child to emerging adult, sometimes angry, funny, silly, excited, or frustrated. I gave her space when she wanted it. She was fifteen.

One evening our family worked together at the dining room table. Dan curled on Cody's lap while she did homework. I paid bills. Dennis idly scratched Milka's ears as he completed an accident report from a minor fender bender. He mentioned he'd just been invited again to Australia and Papua New Guinea for sometime that summer.

Cody asked, "You'll be back for my birthday, right?"

"Of course!" Dennis said.

The relaxed family evening was spent talking and working together, and thinking about birthdays. Four days later, Cody was back at St. Paul Children's Hospital.

I sat in a chair next to her bed. My left arm rested on a pillow with my fingers on Cody's forehead. She said that made her feel more secure when her head hurt. Dennis was at the foot of the bed using the food table as a desk. Cody spoke softly as she drifted in and out of sleep. "I'm just exhausted. Wake me up before surgery. Make me aware, but don't keep me awake or else I'll get cranky." Later she asked, "Why is this happening anyway?" And later, "Oh yeah, this is a game day, isn't it? Hockey. My hockey game is today."

Plastic stickers on Cody's chest held thin wires that monitored her vital signs. An hour before, she'd begun to choke and turned blue. The machine had beeped, but no one was coming. Dennis had yelled, "She's arresting!" I yelled, "She's arresting!"

Dennis grabbed her arm and pulled Cody onto her side. She coughed and started breathing just as the room filled with people. Her chest was a light shade of blue. Those gathered in the room were in high gear, prepared for action. But the need had passed. Dennis was pale and wide-eyed. He had saved our daughter *again*.

The doctor who arrived first told the others, "She's okay. She'd apneaed [stopped breathing] when I came in but began breathing on her own." He instructed someone to put a nasal cannula [plastic tube] with moist oxygen at Cody's nostrils. The clinicians left the room.

Cody said she could hear it happening around her. "I knew I was all right, but I couldn't breathe or talk. I wish I knew CPR, so I could save people."

I asked, "Who would you like to save?"

"Patrick Swayze . . . or Lewis." Cody smiled and closed her eyes again. We went back to waiting. I doodled in a sketchpad. Dennis returned to writing. So far, he'd worked a lot that day, breaking briefly to go for food, then coffee, then save our girl, *again*.

Cody stirred. "You mean I should just calm down and not worry? Did I make a fool of myself? I said something stupid about Lewis. It doesn't matter. I just need reminding to breathe and swallow so I don't choke." She mumbled, "I won't die because I'm too fat, will I? That was another worry I had."

"No, sweetie." I assured her, "You're not fat."

I had once mentioned something I heard about anesthesia being hard on overweight patients—harder to wake up, I think. Cody remembered that before every surgery.

"Mom, definitely tell me what's happening when it happens. I get scared easy. I get scared when no one's holding my hand."

I promised to tell her everything and to keep my hand on her.

I squeezed her fingers gently every once in a while to remind her. I let go for a moment to reach for the phone to call Robbie. She said Art had let out our dogs and she asked how Cody was doing. I agreed to call again when we knew more.

Cody asked, "Can you please put your hand on me?"

I put my hand back on her forehead and stroked her hair. It hadn't grown much since the last surgery. She kept her eyes shut and sighed, "This is what I call scary. I don't like having surgery almost twenty times. What time is this?"

"Eighteen. Eighteen surgeries."

"Mom, could you put your hand on me?"

"It is on you."

Waiting again. Watching and praying that nothing further harmed Cody. The neurosurgeon was unmoved by our concern all day and was operating on someone else. I was afraid to wait this long, afraid of the risk to Cody's eyesight, to her life. I watched her breathe, listened to the click of the IV monitor, and felt the chill of the room.

At 5:30 the sun was setting. My stomach was tight. Dennis turned on the TV to catch the news. Cody was asleep, looking peaceful with her mouth open slightly. The large stuffed beagle Tad gave her for Christmas was cradled under her right arm with the IV tubing. I wrote in my journal: "I'm afraid this time to spend the night with Cody. Two times Dennis found her not breathing; two times he saved her. I'm afraid I won't notice if it happens. What if I fall asleep and don't notice? I don't want her to die. I watch her sleep. She's so beautiful. Her lashes are long; her cheek is pink. Her forehead is moist. She must be warm. I adjust her covers. I stare around the room. I don't want to wait anymore."

Finally, Cody was taken into surgery—*in God's hands now,* I thought. I reminded myself that she's always in God's hands. *I hate fear.*

After surgery I saw that the doctor had allowed a much larger area of Cody's head to be shaved than necessary. She would have some choice words about his heartlessness.

The next day Cody was still unable to look up past the midpoint. A nurse suggested that recovery might take longer now that Cody was older. "Surgeries age a body." I figured my daughter must be older than me by this time.

When I arrived to take Dennis's place the third afternoon, Cody was sitting up, chomping an apple, and listening to The Jets on her boom box. She greeted me, "Mom! I met a very cute boy today with a disease. And, the doctor says I can go home after one more day of IV meds."

Fear was history as Cody looked forward to the evening. Darryl, the "boy with the disease," was going to watch *Dirty Dancing* with her on the VCR that Play Lady put in her room.

At home the next day, Cody began to straighten her room but tired quickly. All weekend, she did nothing but homework and sleep. Frustrated after two hours, she groaned, "What is wrong with me? I thought I was good at math."

Despite how fragile Cody's life seemed at times, she remained a "tough little bugger" as Dennis observed later that night. But I feared there was more to come. Three brain surgeries in seven weeks. *Enough.* I wanted to get back in touch with feelings of joy the way Cody always did.

I invited her to work with me Monday morning. She seemed tired. I wanted to be sure she was strong enough to go back to school. By 10:00 a.m., she had a headache and couldn't look up. Cody hadn't even been out of the hospital long enough to remove stitches from the last surgery, and her shunt was failing again.

Bundled in her winter coat, hat, and gloves, Cody sat limp in her wheelchair with her eyes shut as we entered the hospital and rode the elevator. When the door opened on the third floor, two nurses who knew her stood in the hallway. Both women looked at Cody in disbelief and said, "Not again?!"

Like Jason in *Friday the Thirteenth,* Cody intoned, "I'm ba-aa-ack."

The nurses shook their heads in sympathy and laughed.

Father Dan had already arrived at the hospital. Our priest knew this was a lot of brain surgery in a short period. He dipped his thumb in a small container and rubbed an oily cross on Cody's forehead while he prayed.

Surgery number nineteen was the fourth consecutive brain surgery without finding a problem with the shunt itself. The neurosurgeon admitted being perplexed, but determined to stop the cycle. He showed us CAT scans from before and after surgery. The shunt tip looked pushed into the side of a ventricle in both images. I asked if the position of the shunt might be preventing fluid from draining. He dismissed my question with, "I think it's fixed now."

In two days Cody was again sitting up in her hospital bed, singing to music, moving her shoulders to the beat. Despite her cheeriness, I wasn't sure her shunt was fixed this time, either. Her eyes still wobbled when she tried to look up. I stared at the stuffed beagle on the windowsill. Cody brought it to the hospital again to feel as though her other dad was with her, too. I jotted a reminder in my sketchpad to tell Tad she said that. He was due to call later in the day.

Dennis was coming at noon. I planned to run home, shower, and go to work for a few hours. I wanted to shake the feeling of gloom. *Didn't I used to be better at this?* Cody bobbed her head to the music as she sang. She was chirpy and anxious to be home.

That night Dennis told me, "Cody's spirit is invincible." *It's true,* I thought, *she's rarely depressed, and never for long.* I wondered how she did it.

Cody came home Friday morning, slept all day and awoke with a headache. Cody was scared again, and so was I. Dennis reminded us that the neurosurgeon said it might take weeks for the eye pressure to decrease after so many surgeries within such a short time. I wanted to believe that all was well, but the evidence wasn't there. Cody sounded cheery talking to Tad on the phone later that night.

I wrote in my journal: "If only I could know for sure that she would be okay. I remember Charlie's words about faith. If you know something for sure, then you don't need faith. That's how it works. I pray constantly these days. Faith is hard. Fear is easy."

At an all-day seminar on Saturday, a classmate told me about a forty-five-year-old friend with spina bifida who worked for the State of North Carolina. She assured me, "Cody will be fine."

When I came home, Dennis said Cody slept all day. I went in to check on her. She raised her head from the pillow and her eyes wobbled as she strained to look up at me. "Mom, call the doctor! I didn't want to tell Dennis and make him upset, but my shunt isn't working."

Cody's regular neurosurgeon wasn't available for operation number twenty. His senior partner was on call and would perform the shunt revision. Cody kept her eyes shut, but she listened as the doctor talked. He scribbled notes on a chart as he explained to Dennis and me that there appeared to be no problem with the shunt apparatus itself. He surmised that scar tissue in the abdominal cavity might be preventing fluid from draining. He spoke fast. "This time, we'll direct the shunt tubing through the right jugular vein to Cody's heart."

When I told him she had that type of shunt until age four, the neurosurgeon looked crushed. "The same vein can't be used twice; it would be scarred from the original surgery."

To insert tubing into the jugular vein on the other side required a radiologist and technicians. The full team wasn't available on a Saturday night. The doctor wanted to wait until Monday. Despite our fears about the risk of apnea and blindness with the delay, this physician inspired a bit more confidence than his absent colleague. He was just as gruff and blunt, but he didn't back out of the room while we asked questions.

When this nightmare of uncertainty began two months before and Cody first stopped breathing, the emergency care physician in the PICU was a cardiologist. My letter to the hospital had praised his gentle and professional manner. Dr. Ring worked seven days on and seven days off and looked a bit rumpled whenever we saw him. I was grateful to learn that this was his "on" week. He touched my hand when he spoke with me and seemed to understand how this roller coaster of serious surgeries, and incomplete recoveries, left us in perpetual fear.

On Saturday night I slept on a mat on the floor. The apnea monitor malfunctioned continuously through the night. Cody refused painkillers other than Tylenol. She didn't want to feel dizzy or drowsy. Her pain was so severe that her doctor said it was putting strain on her body. She reluctantly agreed to be given Demerol. The pain didn't go away completely, but she was able to sleep.

On Sunday I sat cross-legged on Cody's hospital bed next to her knees. She lay on her back with her eyes shut and held my hand. Whenever the Demerol wore off, she was miserable and angry, telling me to stop touching her, telling everyone to be quiet. Each sound was loud and shot pain into her head. Nurses tiptoed in and out.

Despite the life-and-death nature of the situation, I began to notice small miracles: Cody's one day at home had allowed us a much-needed break from the hospital. I'd been able to attend a required all-day seminar for my team management class. We'd all slept. We now had the added expertise of the senior partner of the neurosurgery practice. The best people in the PICU, including Dr. Ring, were caring for Cody. When Cody called Charlie for a prayer, he answered on the first ring. I was allowed a mat on the floor in the PICU instead of just a chair, so my neck was not throbbing in pain. By waiting until Monday, Cody's regular neurosurgeon would also be available to participate in the surgery with his senior partner. That felt right.

As I thought more about it, I was also amazed that, despite several short trips, Dennis had not been out of town for any of these five recent surgeries. I couldn't imagine going through this alone with Cody. So far, things were progressing safely. Though my stomach was behaving as usual, acidic and barely functional, I noticed I wasn't scared anymore. God was directing all of it. There was nothing I needed to do, or could do, to influence the results. This was a long list of synchronized miracles.

Dennis felt fragile Sunday night, but I felt faithful. We marveled that one of us stayed strong during each of Cody's emergencies. The role alternated. I didn't know how else we could have endured the stress. We imagined how terrific it would be to have clones to step in for a while. Though the waiting was strenuous, an end was in sight. This complex and serious surgery would work. I was unable to imagine it not working. I let go and left the situation to God.

Awake and alert before surgery Monday morning, Cody said, "Demerol really helped, Mom. I can't believe I was so stupid to be afraid of it. I see why people like this."

Cody said she felt scared for a moment before going into the operating room. We said a prayer, and off she went. I waited out the surgery by myself because Dennis had a meeting. I wasn't scared. I figured this must be how it feels to let God solve problems. I spent the next few hours on a take-home final for my class.

Once Cody was back in her hospital bed, I had no desire to sketch the room or write details in my journal as I often did when she slept after surgery. The crisis was over; she was safe. I called Charlie to thank him for his support and prayers during the two-month nightmare. I made similar calls throughout the evening. I told family and friends that Cody was fine now. Every time I said it, angel shivers confirmed it.

The monitors came off on Tuesday and Cody smiled most of the day, starting when Darryl stopped in to say hello. He looked healthy and was going home. Robbie and Amy visited. Robbie offered to stay the night to give Dennis and me a break. But in truth, the sweet nights with Cody in the hospital during and after life-and-death experiences were the most precious.

Cody improved fast. I was so full of positive faith that I was startled if her eyes quivered or her head drooped in fatigue. I expected her to be 100 percent right away. I told everyone about the combination of miracles involved.

By the time Cody wheeled out of her hospital room to head home, Darryl was readmitted. He'd been home for only two days when sickle cell anemia assaulted him again. He was writhing in pain when we passed his room. We heard him scream and cry that he didn't want another IV.

That night in bed with a dog under each arm, Cody thanked God for all the miracles and said, "It felt so bad to leave when Darryl was so sick and hurting." She said a prayer for Darryl and put her head on her pillow. "You know, Mom, when I told that neurosurgeon I wanted to come home in time for your birthday tomorrow, he said, 'Your mother will have other birthdays.' I was so mad when he said that, I felt red hot."

She let me kiss her.

Chapter 15

Good News

I WOKE UP on my thirty-eighth birthday feeling old, stiff, and achy. So far, 1988 had been an exhausting year and it was only March. In the ten weeks since our Christmas trip east Cody had triumphed over breathing arrests, five brain surgeries, blindness, and gripping fear. Faith won out and I was brought to my knees, grateful for every miracle. Cody was alive, well, and in her own bed.

Until her strength returned, Dennis and I helped with some everyday activities she normally did for herself, such as dressing and climbing into the tub. I washed away remnants of surgical soap from Cody's head and neck without touching the incision. As I helped her pull on a sweatshirt, careful not to touch the surgical staples on her head, Cody said, "I don't even have energy for fun things. Scratch my incision, Mom. It itches."

I used a white cloth to rub the area around her surgery site. I'd removed many stitches, but taking metal staples out of my daughter's head gave me the creeps. I'd let her doctor do that.

Cody was healthy and her weight was good. She'd lost ten pounds in recent months. I cut short what was left of her hair, and she wore scarves or turban-style hats for a few weeks. She went back to the hospital each day of spring vacation to visit Darryl and the other kids. Going back there didn't appeal to me, but I appreciated Cody's kindness to her new friends.

My father stopped in on his way to Spokane on business. In solidarity, he wore a turban and posed for pictures. Dad, Dennis, Cody, and Milka all wore turbans. "You're one tough cookie," Dad told Cody, "I admire you very much." They smiled at each other.

Lewis and Cynthia dropped by with exciting news. They were working on their own Habitat for Humanity house with a goal of moving in by May. Cody, Dennis, and I offered to help, too.

I knew Cody was back to her old self a few days later when she played a joke on Cynthia. Cody called her on April 1st and said, "I have great news. I entered your name in a contest, and I just heard you won—a St. Bernard puppy!" She covered the receiver to giggle.

I pictured Cynthia with a look of horror on her face as Cody continued, "The puppy's arriving tonight on Northwest Airlines, and you need to pick it up at nine o'clock."

Cynthia said, "Okay, well, thank you. Uh, hang on while I get a pencil."

"Wait!" Cody burst out laughing. "April Fools!" Cynthia laughed. She admitted being immensely relieved not to be adopting what would be an enormous dog.

Cody snuggled into her pillow that night and said, "I'm comfy in bed. I haven't been so comfy in a long time." As I leaned down and kissed her cheek, she smiled and said, "Let's plan my birthday!"

"Good idea!" I agreed, "Sixteen is a big deal, and even more important after everything that's happened to you this year."

Cody sat up and said, "Let's have a big party and a talent show! We can tell guests to bring a talent to do in front of everybody."

She called my parents to tell them about her party and learned that my mother also had a big party when she turned sixteen, with a barbeque and games. Cody said, "Then it's a family tradition!" But Mom and Dad were sorry they couldn't come to Cody's party. My father was a ceramics engineer who traveled frequently to cities where large refractories processing kilns he'd invented were in use. A few days before Cody's birthday in August, he had to present a paper in Sydney, Australia. Cody teased, "I'm really sorry, Grandpa, that I won't be able to see you sing and dance in front of all my friends!"

Cody, Dennis, and I worked through April on the Habitat for Humanity house. While Dennis was in New Orleans and Cody was at school, I went on a Thursday to paint a hallway. As I was leaving, a gray-haired man in bib overalls was applying exterior stucco. He stopped to chat. He said he'd worked on 125 different Habitat for Humanity homes. When I told him some family friends were the new homeowners, he asked, "Can white people live in these houses? Are your friends colored or white?"

I said my friends were "black." He asked who else I knew in the organization.

"I know Joel. He's in charge of building this house."

"Oh, is he the head nigger?"

My stomach twisted. The man exchanged wide grins with a younger coworker and chuckled, "You see, I'm from Florida, and down there . . ." He went on about "coloreds" he knew who worked construction. The punch line of his story included the word "nigger" again. The younger man smiled and looked up quickly to see if I appreciated the joke. My cheeks were hot, but I couldn't think of a thing to say! The old man's weathered face creased in a smile as he added, "Those coloreds really laughed at that."

Flustered, I turned and walked quickly to my car. The stucco man called after me, "It was a pleasure meeting you." He didn't have a clue that I was angry. I threw him a disgusted look. The younger man was watching me. I became angrier as I drove away, thinking how ineffectual I'd been. I'd done *nothing* to let the man know how offensive he was.

Cody's bus dropped her off just as I arrived home. I told her about the stucco man. We fumed together for several minutes in our disgust at bigotry. We agreed that, no matter what, it's important to say something to let people like the stucco man know that racist language is unacceptable. We tried to think of things I could have said.

"That isn't funny."

"Your language is offensive."

"That story is offensive."

Cody suggested, "Fuck you, buddy!"

Cody and I spent four hours on Saturday working at the Habitat for Humanity house. I told Joel about the stucco man. Surprised, he said, "I'm sorry I wasn't here. I'm really sorry." He sounded protective of me, but I remained ashamed that I'd said nothing.

While painting the wood trim in a hallway, Cody told me, "Grandma said some odd things at Christmas about black people."

I held the paint can for Cody to dip her brush and asked, "What did she say?"

"I told her how much fun camp was with Lewis there last summer, and Grandma said, 'If you fall for a black man, you'll have black babies.'"

"What did you say?"

"I told her I think babies with dark skin are more beautiful."

"I always thought that, too." I put the paint can on a step stool near Cody.

"Grandma said when she was little, she saw white boys throw dirt on some black children's ice cream cones. She said that same thing could happen to me if I have black friends."

I wiped a dribble of paint from Cody's wheel and told her, "When I was a teenager, Mom told me I should only date people like me, because apples stay with apples, and oranges stay with oranges. But that didn't even make sense. The fruit bowl in Mom's kitchen had apples, oranges, grapefruit, and bananas."

"I told Grandma that I like a person for who they are, and Lewis is my best friend no matter what color he is."

"Good for you, sweetie. Was that the end of it?"

"She told me to just be careful." Shaking her head, Cody said, "I love Grandma, but she's weird."

A story appeared in the *Star Tribune* in mid-May that showed "handicapped youngsters" Cody and Lewis playing tennis as part of a community education program. The picture above the article showed Cody smiling with her racket held high. Lewis's eyes were on the ball just as he was about to whack it. The caption read: "I used to like to watch it when I was little, and never thought I'd be able to do it myself," said Cody, a girl who has spent her entire life in a wheelchair. "I played other sports, soccer and floor hockey, but this is the one I like best."

Cody stayed busy with tennis, school, concerts, fun with "big sister" JP, and sleepovers with girlfriends. As ninth grade came to an end, she heard a rumor about a threatened cutback of teachers at South High that included her favorite teacher, Mr. Debe. She called his home to confirm that the rumor was true, then wrote a letter to each member of the school board and asked to speak at the upcoming meeting. Dennis offered to speak, too.

There was standing room only when the three of us entered the crowded public hearing. School Board members took seats at tables on a raised platform with clusters of microphones. Around the room, people held signs protesting the threatened cutbacks. We waited by the entrance and listened as names were called and people came forward to speak in front of TV cameras. As folks shifted positions, we inched closer to the front.

Cody's name was announced and a microphone was passed to Dennis. He held it as she read her statement in a clear voice: "My name is Cody Cornell. I am a ninth grade student at South High. I would like to say a few words about my feelings about the cutback of teachers. I am especially concerned because a few of my teachers are the ones being cut. One is the teacher who has made the difference for me. Before this year, I didn't do very well in school. I thought all teachers were boring and that school was boring." The crowd laughed.

Cody paused and looked up at the school board members before continuing. "That has all changed since I had Mr. Dennis Debe as a teacher. I think instead of cutting back teachers, we should strongly consider cutting back on other things. Do not cut back great teachers like Mr. Debe." The crowd applauded.

Dennis spoke next and cited demographic information that reinforced the folly of cutting teachers. He concluded with an affirmation of the seriousness of the school board's task in making responsible budget cuts.

The last day of school was three days later. Cody cried before she went to sleep that night, as she did every year when school ended. Her summer job started the next day in the library, putting barcodes on books for the Minneapolis Public Schools.

Within days, Cody heard that Mr. Debe didn't lose his job. We invited him and his wife for a celebratory dinner. Cody was ecstatic to have her favorite teacher come to our house. But after the Debes left she told me she'd become panicky at dinner. She had tickled Mr. Debe's knee under the table for several seconds before realizing she wasn't touching her own knee. She had excused herself for a few moments to go to her room.

"It made me so nervous, Mom; I had to listen to music to calm down."
If Mr. Debe noticed, he didn't say so.

As the date of the Cody's birthday celebration approached, party details
fell into place. Since our house was small, we decided to hold the event in
the social hall at St. Albert's Church.

Cody screamed, "Yippee!" when my brother Charlie called to say that he
and Zachary were driving from St. Louis to attend the celebration. Zach, at
eleven, was a natural entertainer. He planned to impersonate Elvis Presley.

Cody decided to sing a song from *Annie*. She asked Dennis and me to
sing a duet of the mouse song from *Cinderella*. Tad and I used to sing it
in rapid falsetto voices when Cody was small. Since Tad couldn't come to
the party, Cody asked Dennis to learn the mouse song. She laughed hard
when he practiced. His Australian accent made the falsetto even funnier.

Cody wrote home from camp in late July:

Dear Mom,
Michelle and I have our own room. There's a cute guy here. He's in a wheel-
chair. He asked me to dance, and I said yes. That was after being too shy to
dance with anyone and turning down half a dozen guys before him. God got
a hold of me and said, go ahead try out not being shy. Michelle and I love
to do the same things. I can't wait to see Dan and Milka. Say hi to Dad and
don't forget to bring Amy and the dogs when you come get me. Well, see ya!!
Love, Cody
*   P.S. I love and miss you all. (Only a month and three days.)*

Dennis left for two weeks in Papua New Guinea and Australia. He'd visit
his mother and return the day of the big party. Dennis was nervous as
usual about air travel. Cody hugged and kissed him before he got out
of the car at the airport. Once he was gone, she started to cry. "I worry
about Dad. He's a wimp like me. He gets scared. I'm afraid something
terrible could happen to him."

"Honey, your dad travels all the time. He's smart. He can take care of
himself. But if you want, we can call him in Australia when he gets to his
mother's house."

We stopped on the way home to buy Elmer's glue, glitter, and an oversized white T-shirt for Cody to wear like a dress over silver stretch pants at her birthday party. We spread the shirt on the dining room table and used five colors of glitter to make designs. As Cody applied sparkles in designated areas, she said, "I don't want Dad to miss my birthday."

I assured her, "He won't."

I drew a giant "16" in glue below the neckline of the shirt. Cody sprinkled pink glitter on the glue. She smiled and said, "I think Dad is cute. But don't tell him I said that." She drew swirls and stars in glue and added silver, blue, and green glitter.

"This is beautiful, sweetie. You're going to look gorgeous in this."

Cody looked at the shirt, smiled, and made her three-syllable squeal.

Two days before the party, Cody called me at work, sobbing. "Uncle Charlie called. Grandpa had a heart attack when he got to Australia!"

My stomach churned the way it did during Cody's medical emergencies. I knew Mom must be scared. I phoned Dennis at his mother's house in Fairy Meadow. He called the Sydney hospital and located Mom. Dad was being monitored, but there was no definitive information about his condition. So far, *thank God*, at least my father was alive.

Cody observed, "It's a miracle that Dad was still in Australia to help Grandma."

I felt angel shivers.

The phone rang early Saturday morning. My father was in stable condition, and Dennis's mother had gone to Sydney to be with Mom.

Cody screamed, "Yaaaay! That's the best way to start my birthday!"

She stayed by the phone while I picked up her cake and went to the airport to meet Dennis's plane. By the time Charlie and Zach arrived in the afternoon, Cody was dressed in her birthday glitter. Party time!

Fifty guests attended the Cody Cornell 16th Birthday Party and Talent Show: friends, neighbors, the Debes, Father Dan, and others. The social hall at St. Albert's was decorated with streamers and dozens of helium-filled balloons. The food was delicious and laughter was continuous.

Lewis did a drum roll as each talent was introduced. Some families did skits together, and performers as young as three sang songs and danced. Cody's attendant from school presented her with a special recognition certificate for her part in putting barcodes on 80,000 library books. Dennis and I wore mouse ears and sang our silly song. Zach wore a shiny red shirt, played guitar, and gyrated as Elvis.

Cody was the last performer. After she sang *Maybe*, the crowd erupted in applause. She unfolded a piece of paper and read, "I would like to say a few words and dedicate a song to someone special. Today, as we all know, is my birthday. Eight months ago, I wondered if I would even have a birthday this year because, as most of us know, I was in the hospital and had five very serious operations. I stopped breathing twice. I owe my life and today to a lot of people, God, and all the people who were praying for me. But I especially owe my life to the man who caught me not breathing both of those times that I stopped—the one extra special man in my life, the man who I'm very proud to call my dad. Thanks to my dad, I didn't die young. So here is one of my favorite songs, and it's dedicated to my dad."

As James Taylor's *Never Die Young* began to play, Cody asked Dennis to dance. Smiles and tears were on the faces of our friends as Dennis kissed Cody and spun her around the dance floor.

When the party was over, Cody, Zach, Amy, and Lewis left St. Albert's together, holding onto a huge bunch of balloons. The summer had been a scorcher, but there was a balmy breeze that evening. Laughing continued as the group discussed the performances and walked the ten blocks home.

Later in bed, Dennis and I talked about how precious and poised Cody was as she sang and gave her speech. Dennis hadn't known she planned a dedication to him. He laughed and said, "When she began speaking, I assumed she was about to thank Mr. Debe for something."

The good-time glow lasted among Cody's friends. Lewis rode his bike over to our house a few times before school started. A week later Dad was well enough to fly home from Australia. He would need quintuple bypass surgery once he was stronger.

Summer heat extended through most of September. The news reported that forty percent of Yellowstone Park burned away. Fires continued to roar out of control. The wind was hot in our neighborhood and leaves were dry on the trees. Cody developed a low-grade fever, headache, and bladder infection that lasted several days just as Dennis left for Japan. Cody looked at me with a worried expression. A bladder infection was a normal type of problem for her, easily treated. But this time, after all that had happened so recently, we both overreacted. I felt her fear, and my own. Her illness, in combination with the oppressive heat and gruesome news reports, caught me in a haze of gloomy thoughts. We said a short prayer; I kissed her and suggested she take a nap.

The news was packed with stories about bigotry, medical waste strewn across beaches, crack houses in family neighborhoods, mothers offering their children to be fondled in exchange for drugs. I cringed at humanity's arrogant use of the earth—the fragile ozone layer, diminishing rainforests. Thoughts of rage and distress for the innocent grabbed me like a crackling arm reaching out of the heat. My heart ached for the displaced wildlife, hospitalized babies, abused children and animals. I felt ashamed to let these things batter me down. *I have to change my thoughts.* I reminded myself to put Cody back in God's hands, again. Again, it was hard. I had to remember that there was still hope and honor, people who care, and true selfless love.

I watered each thirsty houseplant, wiped the leaves with a damp towel, and checked on Cody. She was asleep with her head resting on her stuffed beagle and her arm around Milka. Her forehead was cool now. I breathed a prayer of thanks.

Chapter 16

Blue, Sex, and Action

In mid-October I was working on a series of paintings when Cody called from school. "Mom, you have to come here now. You won't believe the dog that's here. I'm waiting for the bus to go play hockey. Please come, Mom. He doesn't have a collar, he's thin, and he's the smartest dog I ever saw."

"Cody, I'm so busy right now. He probably lives in that neighborhood."

"Please, Mom, this dog is special. I don't think he has a family. Please? The bus will be here any second. I'll have to go."

"Okay, babe." I dropped my brushes in a pot of water and put the fresh-squeezed globs of acrylic paint in the freezer. South High was only five minutes away.

The schoolyard was empty when I arrived—except for the adaptive hockey team. Nine players stood in a line, waiting for the bus. I noticed some new kids this year. Cody was the only one in a wheelchair.

"Mom, watch this." A medium-sized black dog ran from the field and dropped a stick in front of a boy wearing an ankle brace. The dog stepped back, crouched in play position, and waited. The boy tossed the stick. The dog brought it back and put it at the feet of a boy in a helmet. He threw the stick, and the dog brought it to the feet of the next kid. This continued until the dog came to Cody. He put a paw on her footrest and gently dropped the stick on her lap.

"See, Mom? See how smart he is? He's so sweet!"

The bus arrived just as Cody threw the stick. She rolled onto the wheelchair lift and into the bus. The attentive black dog dropped his stick at my feet and waited. I tossed it as I scanned the area for anyone who might recognize him. I walked one way, then the other. The dog stayed close, coaxing me to throw his stick again.

I decided to ignore him and walk to my car. As I opened the car door, he raced past me, jumped in, and sat in the passenger seat, facing forward, ready to go.

At home, after friendly sniffing with Milka and Dan, he wandered through the house. When he perched on his hind legs to look at individual paintings on the walls, I was dumbfounded.

When Cody came home from school, the dog raced to greet her and put his front paws in her lap. She hugged him and said, "He looks like a big Milka or a giant Dan." He looked so similar to our dogs; we assumed he was a cockapoo. That's how I listed him on the "found dog" notices. Cody said, "I wish we could keep him, Mom. He's so smart!"

"A dog this terrific is probably somebody's best friend."

She begged, "If nobody claims him, can we please keep him?"

I said, "We'll see. Three dogs . . . is a lot of dogs."

I called the pound weekly and scanned the newspaper for lost-dog notices. Two weeks later, I read: Lost: Black Cockapoo, female, etc. I was so relieved to see "female," I realized I wanted to keep the dog, too. Dennis named him Blue.

Dennis, Cody, and I flew to Pittsburgh at Thanksgiving to see my father after his heart surgery. Cody sat with Dad and we all tried to keep him comfortable.

We rented a car for a quick trip to Philadelphia. Cody saw her former teacher, Mrs. R, and contacted her old boyfriend, Ryan. We spent an evening with my friend Jackie and her teenage son, Lee. On the plane home Cody said, "Let's move back to Philly. There's good music on the radio, good friends, and cute boys."

Days later, Cody had a bad headache. We figured it was from uncomfortable beds on our trip, but when the pain worsened we were directed to the emergency room. We stopped on the way to the hospital for a chiropractic adjustment to Cody's neck, just in case.

In the ER, tears streamed down her cheeks as surgery was arranged.

Cody said, "I'm only afraid of three things: looking stupid in hats to cover my shaved head, death, and apnea."

Her use of the word "only" and her grouping together of hair loss, death, and apnea made me laugh. She laughed, too.

Dennis, Cody, and I said a prayer together for complete healing and, within an hour, all shunt problem symptoms disappeared. The neuro-surgeon sent Cody home. Despite such a marvelous miracle, the initial panic Cody experienced during this emergency stuck with her for several days. She suggested, "Maybe I should go see Dick."

Dick was a marriage counselor Dennis and I had seen a few years before. I'd recently begun seeing him again. He arranged for a female colleague to help Cody deal with the realistic fears in her life and for her life. Cody said she liked having her own therapist.

After Dennis spent most of January in Australia he initiated talk about our moving to Oz after Cody finished high school. She didn't like that idea. He discussed it further with her while I visited friends one week-end in March. Cody's voice quivered the night I returned home. "I told Dad I don't want to move to Australia. I don't want to be so far from my friends. But he kept trying to convince me. I don't know if I'm even safe there. I have to know there are good enough doctors and hospitals in case I need surgery."

I assured her, "No one will force you to move to Australia. And we won't move anywhere that doesn't have excellent medical care for you."

Dennis was reading in bed when I brought up Cody's concerns. He lowered his book and said, "By the time we move to Oz, Cody will be eighteen. She'll be able to live on her own; she doesn't have to come. The long flight and quarantine regulations are too much for the dogs anyway. They can stay here with her." My heart began to beat a little faster.

I told Dennis, "I don't want to live that far from Cody or the dogs. If she had a medical emergency, it would take too long to get to her. She always needs an advocate. You know bad things happen in hospitals."

"She's only in tenth grade. There's time to think about it." He went back to his book.

The idea of living in Australia without Cody or the dogs horrified me.

I hoped my husband would change his mind by the time Cody finished high school. I wasn't sure what I'd do if he didn't. I couldn't imagine living so far from Cody. I looked over at Milka curled in her pink dog bed. Dan lay next to me, licking his paw. Blue was asleep beside him. Each dog was a treasure—for me and for Cody. I put thoughts about a move to Australia out of my mind.

A few days later Dennis was in Baltimore. I was reading in bed when Cody came into the room and said, "I think I do have an ulcer. I feel better with those pills."

She'd started a prescribed antacid medication for frequent stomachaches. I asked her to tell me more about what things made her nervous.

"I get too shy around boys I like. I don't know what to say."

"You can talk to boys who are friends, right?"

"That's different."

"The best way to get to know a boy you like is to be friends. Even if it doesn't become romantic, you still have a friend, right?"

"I'm friends with Lewis and I like him as a boyfriend, too. But he has another girlfriend. He makes me so mad. He treats me weird at school sometimes. I'm afraid I'll never have another *real* boyfriend again, like Ryan."

"You were *seven* when Ryan was your boyfriend. Being a teenager is more complicated."

"Tell me about it!" Cody rolled her eyes and smiled. She asked, "Is there any reason I can't have babies?"

"You can get pregnant the same way anyone does. Some things might be harder to do while you're pregnant since you can't walk. I don't know what it'd be like for you to give birth. It might be hard to push a baby out. But you could have a cesarean where the doctor makes an incision in your tummy to get to the baby."

"No surgery," Cody said. "I've had enough surgeries."

"I really don't know enough about it, honey. But we can find out more. We'll ask a doctor. We need to find some older women in wheelchairs, so you can ask them how they handle boyfriends and sex. Maybe you could get some tips."

"Mom! You can't just ask people how they have sex!" We both laughed.

"Okay, we'll find some books or videos about relationships and sex for people with disabilities." Cody liked that idea.

The next day I began calling libraries, advocacy organizations, and the human sexuality program at the University. I made calls all over the country, following a trail of referrals, and found little to help Cody. I ordered books on sexuality for people with disabilities. Cody and I were disappointed to find that each book focused primarily on paralyzed men, penile implants and pumps. There was scarcely anything about sex for women with disabilities. A few books mentioned that a sense of humor was helpful during sex when one or both partners have disabilities, especially if incontinence was a factor. There was no guarantee that a person wouldn't pee at the wrong time. Being squeamish about bodily functions could hamper the experience.

Two of my girlfriends had physical disabilities, but neither was in a wheelchair. Neither knew of any helpful materials or books on sex. One friend told me, "The first guy I had sex with wanted me on top. I couldn't hold myself up in that position; I was horribly embarrassed. I could've used a book like the one you're looking for."

I called a local nonprofit support organization for parents of children with disabilities. The woman I spoke with apologized. She said that members of their group preferred to think of their children as "asexual." "Many of our parents are afraid that sex is not in the cards for their handicapped child anyway. It's a messy topic."

Cody and I kept talking and reading, and studying materials we found. We both grew increasingly frustrated and angry that resources focused only on men. Cody's sensitivity to discrimination against women intensified as she noticed sexist language in magazines and TV ads. She pointed out to me when she heard someone make a sexist comment. She asked me to buy her a *Playgirl* magazine.

As Cody became more attuned to issues of fairness, she spoke up when confronted with barriers. If a store was not accessible for a person in a wheelchair, Cody asked to talk to someone in charge to voice a complaint. When she ordered tickets by phone for a concert, a ticket agent repeated back, "So you need tickets for two people and a wheelchair?"

Tired of being referred to as "a chair," Cody firmly repeated, "No, I need three tickets, and one will be used by a *person* in a wheelchair."

The ticket agent repeated, "Right, two regular tickets and one chair. The wheelchair will be in the handicapped section, and the two people will sit in the row behind the chair."

Cody argued in frustration, "I want to sit with my parents, not in front of them."

I took the phone. "Look, my husband and I want to take our daughter to this concert as a special occasion. We want to sit together, enjoy the concert *together*. Can that happen?"

The best we accomplished was one folding chair next to Cody in the handicapped section. Due to the inflexibility she encountered buying tickets, Cody often attended concerts with friends with disabilities rather than with those who couldn't sit with her.

Cody's interest in and concerns about sex prompted me to visit the adult section of a video store. I hoped to find something educational that addressed sexuality for people with disabilities, something that provided sex information without being pornographic. Dennis came with me. We scanned shelves, looking for films made by academic institutions. Video jackets showed photos of balloon-sized breasts and couples in erotic poses. I was ready to give up when I found a video narrated by a family therapist claiming to demonstrate sexuality for "normal" married couples. I told Cody, "We couldn't find anything about sex and disability, but we rented a video that shows a couple having sex. Do you want to watch it?" She said okay.

Dennis turned on the VCR. The film began with a discussion of "normal and natural, healthy sexuality between a loving husband and wife." The narrator said, "It is perfectly fine to try different positions while having sexual relations." She stressed that anything a couple finds comfortable, and does not cause harm, is appropriate during sex. The "husband and wife" appeared to be having intercourse, demonstrating a variety of positions. Oral sex was described as a "nice" alternative that did not risk pregnancy. Nothing the couple did conveyed even the slightest hint of passion. Far from pornographic, the portrayal was so antiseptic that sex came across as unnatural and robotic. After ten minutes, Cody turned around and said, "Do you mind if I stop watching this? I think I might throw up."

"Thank you!" Dennis responded and turned off the VCR.

I burst out laughing, "I'm sorry, honey. That was pretty terrible."

When school was finished in June, I joined Dennis on a business trip to Vancouver. Amy and Kari stayed with Cody. The girls promised to be responsible, share meal preparation, and care for the dogs. Robbie offered to be available in case of emergency. I called home the first night and Cody cheerfully told me how the dogs were. I asked about her first day of work.

She said, "I don't know if I want this summer job." She described each thing she did at work, and how some of it was hard. Sighing, she said, "I don't think I can do it."

"It's just the first day, babe. Take your time. You'll get the hang of it."

Cody interrupted, "We might go to Norma Jean's on Tuesday night. We want to go to a real night club and listen to music."

I cautioned, "Teenagers might not be allowed without an adult, honey. It's a bar."

She said, "We'll call and find out. I hope we can go."

I was relieved that Cody was fine. I'd found it hard not to worry about her over the past year. Not knowing when another medical emergency might occur was sometimes a strangulating threat. After I hung up, I told Dennis, "I need to shed this worried feeling, but I forget how."

Dennis said, "She's fine. She'll be fine."

"I know. *She's* not the burden. These *feelings* are the burden."

A few weeks after we came home, Cody decided to take Dennis's last name. When he adopted Cody, Dennis didn't think it necessary to change her name from Cornell to Ahlburg. She had toyed with the idea before, but now she was sure. "Dad saved my life, Mom."

A lawyer friend started the process. Cody wrote a letter explaining her decision to Tad. She revised it several times before sending it. When she went to camp in July she registered as Cody Ahlburg. When she called home she said, "Camp is boring; I don't want to come back next year. I learned how to transfer from the floor to the camp bed—and it's higher than my bed at home!" Almost an afterthought, she added, "I like it that everyone here calls me Cody Ahlburg."

In a letter from camp she wrote, "I don't miss you, but I love you. I thought I had feeling in my foot today, but it went away, rats! I don't mind being away from home, but I wish I was away from home somewhere else, like in the arms of a certain young guy." She was referring to my friend Jackie's son in Philadelphia. A homemade calendar in Cody's room had a picture of Lee on every month.

After turning seventeen, Cody began St. Albert's confirmation classes, which were held in a building that was not wheelchair accessible. The priest in charge of the classes, Father Tom, made sure Cody was safely lifted in and out of the building, but she was more and more uncomfortable with the arrangement. A weekend retreat was scheduled in another inaccessible location. Cody wrote a letter to Father Tom, explaining her decision not to attend.

> September 22, 1989
>
> Dear Tom,
>
> I originally planned to write to inform you that I have another commitment the weekend of our retreat. I don't have that commitment anymore. But as I was considering this other weekend school trip, it got me to thinking. I don't really feel my needs to feel safe and to feel independent are being met. I think that the meetings and retreats could be held somewhere other than places I can't get to or around in completely, so that I, or anyone else in a wheelchair, could spend the night and do things like everyone else.
>
> Maybe I do have a father and mother who can get me up a few stairs, and do other extra things, but not everybody in a wheelchair has someone to do that for them. I don't feel safe in situations where I can't take care of myself completely. So this is why I've decided not to go on any retreats unless it is to a place where I can stay the whole time like everyone else. I know that you have been trying to make exceptions for me, and trying to fit me in. I appreciate what you have done. It's just

that all my life, I've had exceptions made for me. I want to be treated like everyone else, and do everything like them too. So that's the reason I won't be going on the retreat after all. My mom says to keep the money even if someone else goes in my place.

I would like you to accept this letter as my October 1st report about a social justice issue. The problem I see is that people with disabilities are being excluded from St. Albert's Confirmation Program.

The solutions I propose are: Hold the meetings in places that are fully accessible to everyone. Do not plan an important activity that excludes a disabled person from full participation. Do whatever is possible to make a disabled person feel as important as anyone else.

What I learned is that even people with very good intentions who try to include a disabled person can make the person feel left out without realizing it. I also learned that disabled people have to stick up for their rights every day.

Sincerely,

Cody Ahlburg

The church service that Sunday was held outdoors in nearby Brackett Field. After the service Father Tom came straight over to Cody and thanked her for her letter. He told her she was right; the confirmation program was being moved to an accessible location. Cody gave Tom a shy smile and said, "Cool. Thanks."

At home later, Cody said, "Mom, I want to buy you a suit."

"Sweetie, suits are expensive; save your money." I was starting a half-time job working with psychiatrists in a hospital, and my new position required business attire.

"Mom, I've noticed over the years that you spoil me; you give me a lot. I seriously want to buy some clothes for your new job. I have lots of savings from my birthday and Christmas money, and my summer jobs."

"Okay, then, thank you." I kissed her and said, "Let's go shopping!"

Cody sang in a choir concert the evening of my first day in the new job. I wore the knit suit she bought for me. Cody was the only singer in a wheelchair. She looked beautiful in the spotlight in her blue choir robe.

After thirty hours of prerequisite classroom instruction at a driving school, Cody was ready for behind-the-wheel lessons. A nearby resource center for people with disabilities provided lessons in cars equipped with hand controls. On the day of Cody's final lesson, the teacher invited me to ride along in the backseat.

Cody followed the rules of the road, but slowed almost to a stop a few hundred yards before any intersection. The teacher prompted her to keep going, but Cody hesitated. When Cody turned her head, she also turned the wheel. My heart jumped to my throat a few times on that short trip.

When Cody was little, she sat on my lap and pretended to drive the car. I controlled the gas and brakes as we drove up and down a driveway or in an empty parking lot. If we came close to an obstacle, I'd say, "Whoa! Whoa!" and Cody shrieked with laughter. Now, Cody said she felt nervous driving.

I suggested, "We can't afford a car with hand controls yet anyway. When we can, we'll go to a big parking lot and practice, practice, practice." We were both okay with that idea.

At the Homecoming Pep Fest at Cody's high school, a caged young tiger was paraded through the gym in front of 1,500 cheering students. Cody was appalled to see the frightened animal cower in the small cage. She wrote to the principal. "It is extremely mean to bring an animal locked in a cage so it can't hide or protect itself from a whole bunch of screaming people. Mr. Lewis, we are all animals, and I care deeply for the four-legged ones in this world. I do not like seeing them suffer and put through that fear."

Another version of the same message from Cody was published as a letter to the editor in the student newspaper. She then invited me to her civics class to make a presentation with her on animal exploitation. She had arranged for us to do a similar program the previous spring.

Doing things like that with my daughter caused me to reflect on activities I did as a child with my mother. The only special thing I remembered doing alone with Mom was seeing the movie *Old Yeller* when I was seven. I decided to do more memorable things with Cody. I asked, "Where would you like to go, just us, on a mother-daughter trip?"

Without pausing she said, "Disney World!"

I updated Cody's health summary and identified a hospital in Orlando with the best pediatric neurosurgeons in case of a shunt emergency during our getaway. Then Cody and I had a nonstop four-day vacation in Disney World.

Our only problem occurred the day we arrived. A wheelchair didn't fit in the bathroom of the "handicapped accessible" room at our motel two miles from Disney World. And the sidewalk in front of the room entrances had no curb cuts. We were moved to a different room, but the new room's bathroom didn't accommodate a wheelchair, either. Cody had to transfer to the floor to scoot-crawl into the bathroom to bathe each morning.

At MGM studios we wore sombreros and sang "Groovy Kind of Love." We dressed as rock stars for a *Rolling Stone* magazine cover. We watched a TV show taping, a stage show, and saw how special effects were created for movies. All in all, it was a chummy time.

Cody said she noticed how different it would have been had Dennis come along. We would've seen different exhibits and not visited as many gift shops or food carts. A big difference for me was doing *all* the lifting of her wheelchair in and out of the rental car and maneuvering in first-aid stations and bathrooms. Though hard on my neck, the fun Cody had was worth it. She said, "Neither of us yelled or got upset about anything."

Cody wrote a full summary of our trip in her journal and noted, "I think it's a good idea for mothers and daughters, and fathers and sons, to do things and go places together. I think Mom and I should do this every year. Even though my mom gets crabby sometimes, she is wonderful all the time. I'm noticing as I'm getting older that she's a great and understanding friend and mom. Well, that concludes my trip with Mom."

She told Dennis, "Next time, we should all go to Disney World, Dad. You'd like it."

Chapter 17

The Storm Before the Calm

AT AN APPOINTMENT soon after our mother/daughter trip, Cody's neurosurgeon expressed concern about the short duration between the onset of her symptoms of a shunt problem and the potential for apnea or retinal hemorrhaging. A surgery called a "cervico-medullary decompression" involved removing part of the top neck vertebrae to make more room for Cody's brain stem when there was increased intracranial pressure. Widening the window of available time before a shunt revision surgery could make a shunt breakdown less dangerous.

In light of the incidents with apnea and vision loss two years before, Cody found the recommendation reasonable. The operation was less scary in that it was not an emergency, but recovery was slower. When Cody went back to school on a Monday, she came home worn out. I kept her home the rest of the week. She had a ticket to a Janet Jackson concert on Thursday and I hoped she'd be well enough to attend.

"I feel like I'm getting away with murder," Cody said on Thursday. "I feel guilty going to see Janet Jackson when I didn't go to school."

I assured her, "If you'd gone to school, you'd be too exhausted to go to the concert. You deserve a good time."

"What if I see someone I know at the concert?"

"It's okay, honey. I'm your mother, and I say you can go."

While Cody was at the concert, Dennis called from a hotel in Boston. I told him how exhausted I felt from my new job, hospitals, Cody's long recovery, and an art show deadline.

He made me laugh by reminding me, "You only have two tits."

When Cody came home that night, she said she'd run into two girls from school on the bus. "My stomach turned, Mom! I told them I felt guilty missing school, but my mom knows I love Janet Jackson and she let me."

Cody chatted excitedly about the concert as she got ready for bed. Once in bed she worried, "I haven't heard from Tad in months, Mom. What if he died?"

She had tried to reach Tad by phone to tell him about her surgery, but his phone was disconnected. It was highly unusual not to be in contact with Tad for this long. With so much happening, I hadn't actually noticed that months had gone by since our last contact. Cody sent him a letter and within a week Tad called. She told him about her surgery.

He asked her about school and boyfriends before telling her the reason he'd been out of touch for so long. He'd been the victim of a violent crime.

"What?" Cody asked in horror, "Are you okay, Daddy?"

"I'm fine now. I'm back in Philly."

"Poor Daddy!" Cody handed me the phone.

A former client had assaulted and robbed Tad at his home in Houston. The teenager was likely on drugs and didn't seem to recognize Tad during the assault. He smashed Tad in the head with a hammer and left him bound and bleeding under a blanket.

After the attack Tad was unable to concentrate and had to resign from his social service job. He couldn't speak about the experience for some time. After a few difficult months and some assistance from a victims' organization, he moved back to Philadelphia. He was now supervising the staff for group homes with the same organization where he'd been director of the school for "severely and profoundly retarded" adults.

Cody and I were at once horrified and relieved at Tad's news. She called him every few days to be sure he was still okay.

Cody was tested at school in April to determine vocational interests. Included were more IQ tests. Dennis and I were again told how amazing it was that Cody was doing so well in eleventh grade. She was described as a "cheerful, outgoing, and well-intentioned but naïve young woman who is basically a concrete, simplistic thinker." The report concluded,

"One is at a loss to explain how she has been able to maintain at or near grade-level academic skill acquisition while displaying developmental delays in other verbal, memory, and perceptual motor areas."

As one example of her "deficiency," the report noted that Cody couldn't answer how many days in a year or which direction the sun set. Considering all the things Cody needed to think about just to take care of herself, it struck me that knowing how many days were in a year, or which direction the sun set, was of little consequence.

In a call to my parents, Mom mentioned that my father was in the hospital. She was vague about why, saying something about tests. Cody and Dennis sat close to the phone and tried to listen when I called Dad to ask why he was in a hospital.

He responded, "Did you talk to your mother?"

"Yeah, she just said tests."

Dad spoke slowly. "Elma is reluctant to say the bad words. I have prostate cancer. It's pretty grim."

"Oh, no," I said just as Cody said, "Poor Grandpa!"

Dad went on, "I had a biopsy last week. They said I didn't need an operation. I went home, but this week I was in some bad pain. They admitted me to see if it spread anywhere else. I was poked in all my orifices."

"That's terrible, Dad. Why didn't you tell me about this?"

"I didn't mean to keep it a secret. But I didn't want to make a big deal about it, either. The pain is easily controlled. I'm on Tylenol with codeine now. I'm amazed at how calm I am."

"Oh, Dad."

He continued, "Everybody's gotta die sometime. I never thought I was an exception to that. The disease is not unusual or scary. This may sound out of character, but I'm reading the *Book of John* and finding it very comforting—the King James Version."

That didn't surprise me. Dad always kept a Bible by his bed.

I asked, "Were you freaked out when they told you?"

"I experienced about ten minutes of confusion. But I realized there was no logic in it."

"That's amazing, Dad. I'm proud of you."

Cody chimed in, "That's where I get it!"

I repeated her remark to Dad, and he said, "My goal is to handle myself as well as Cody does in the face of such possibilities and fears."

As I repeated Dad's comment to Cody, he added, "I really mean that."

"I love you, Dad. I'll call you again tomorrow." Cody and Dennis said goodbye together into the phone.

Dad said, "I don't expect any new news by then."

"I'll call even if there's no news."

"I love you, Grandpa!" Cody shouted as I hung up the phone.

Dad went back to work despite his new diagnosis. Although long past retirement age, he enjoyed work and planned to continue as long as he could. He said, "That's an advantage of being your own boss."

One afternoon in May, a man in a wheelchair came toward me on the sidewalk as I swept our front steps. We exchanged hellos. He said he'd seen me before with Cody when she practiced "popping wheelies" to access curbs that didn't have curb cuts.

Cody was afraid to pop wheelies after the time she flipped backwards, so I stood behind her when she practiced on our street corner. She pulled back sharply on the top of her wheels so that the small front wheels lifted off the ground. In the same motion, she propelled forward so the front wheels landed on the curb. With a final thrust, she rolled up onto the curb.

The man told me about his disability and said his wife was also in a wheelchair. I told him that Cody was seventeen—finishing her junior year in high school. I asked if he knew of any organizations she could join to meet female role models. He said the Metropolitan Center for Independent Living (MCIL) in St. Paul provided peer mentors for young people with disabilities. We exchanged phone numbers before he wheeled off.

The woman I spoke with at MCIL said the group's mission was to empower people with disabilities to live independently. An interview was conducted to match Cody with a peer mentor. This was how she met one of her closest friends.

Sharon was almost thirty at the time and used a motorized chair due to cerebral palsy. She could stand, but not steadily, and I had to listen carefully to understand her speech. She lived in her own apartment and had a busy life. She took her peer mentor role seriously and planned regular activities to give Cody opportunities to try new things.

Cody finally was able to talk with an adult woman in a wheelchair about boys and sex.

Cody's summer library job was interrupted by another shunt surgery. The cervico-medullary decompression achieved what it was meant to do: the symptoms of a shunt breakdown progressed more slowly. However, all other fears associated with an emergency brain surgery remained. An advantage from Cody's perspective was that the neurosurgeon on call this time was a woman. Dr. Dunn told us she'd assisted with the cervico-medullary decompression surgery three months earlier. Cody said, "Cool. Then you already know my brain!"

Cody went right back to work after surgery and, at the end of June, Dennis and I left for a conference in Greece. Cody stayed at home with an older friend, Regina. Robbie had copies of Cody's medical summary in case of emergency.

On my first call home Cody reported, "I remembered to give the dogs their heartworm pills, and Regina and I went to a barbeque. We had fun." She listed all the friends and relatives who called her. I felt good knowing so many people were keeping tabs on her.

When I called Cody two days before our flight home, she was full of news about her plans to attend a New Kids on the Block concert that night. She recounted the steps she took to sort out her plans: "I called the Red Cross, Gillette, and the concert people about accessibility and bathrooms. I got a Foley cath, so I don't have to mess with an inaccessible bathroom stall. Sharon and Debbie are both coming with me."

"Wow, babe, you thought of everything. I hope you have a great time!"

I was impressed with her ingenuity. I could tell Cody felt good about it, too.

"Guess what, Mom? I saw that the prize in the Mrs. Minnesota contest is a mink coat! I called Vonnie at the Animal Rights Coalition to see if we can start a protest."

"Great, sweetie! Hey, make sure you're polite and thank anyone who's helping you."

"I am. I will."

Before dinner on the final night of our trip, the phone rang in our room. It was Robbie. "Everything's under control and Cody's safe, but we're at the hospital. It's her shunt."

Robbie conveyed a calm I wished I could feel as she gave further details. Dr. Dunn thought the short time since the last surgery indicated a possible infection around the shunt tubing. Cody was feeling better after a "shunt tap" that removed some cerebrospinal fluid. She was now on antibiotics and could go home. Hopefully the situation would remain stable and Cody could see her regular neurosurgeon at his clinic on Monday. Robbie handed the phone to Cody.

She cried, "I'm scared, Mommy."

Keeping my own fear in check I said, "It's okay, sweetie. Robbie's there and our plane leaves in the morning. You feel safe with Robbie, right?"

Cody said, "Yes, I do." Dennis spoke to Cody; then I said a prayer with her. She repeated, "I feel safe with Robbie."

I felt helpless being so far away but I realized that, even if Dennis and I were home, this situation would be hard, waiting and dreading the worst. *Please, God, keep her safe.*

Dennis and I went to dinner but, true to form, my digestion shut down. I said to Dennis, "This is too much. The options here are so awful. Either she lives with ongoing scary and painful experiences like this, or she dies, and we all lose."

Dennis said, "We ought to find some way to get help for us and Cody for dealing with these chronic problems, this life and death, the ongoing stress."

I decided, "We just have to get through the next twenty-four to forty-eight hours, and deal with whatever happens when we get home." *Please, God, protect all of us.*

I called Cody from the Athens airport in the morning. It was evening in Minneapolis and she had slept on and off all day. Her headache had come back, and Robbie gave her aspirin. Cody sounded groggy but said she felt better.

"I'll call the minute we land in New York."

"Okay, Mom, I love you."

"I love you, babe. Let's say a quick prayer. Dear God, please keep Cody safe and healthy, in Jesus name, amen. Bye, honey."

"Bye, Mom."

I felt awful. I prayed Cody would sleep peacefully with no problems. *Please, God! If only my stomach would settle down.* I reminded myself that I could do no more at home at the moment than I could where I was.

On the plane the pilot announced an unplanned stop in Madrid to pick up more passengers. Our flight would be delayed another three or four hours! Then we were told we wouldn't take off for an *extra* forty minutes. *Aghhhh!* I wanted to scream in frustration. I tried to read, but scanned the same paragraph over and over. Each takeoff and landing was delayed. I doubted that anyone else on the airplane felt such urgency. Others complained about minor inconveniences. One woman whined about her headset to a flight attendant who twice brought her a new set.

I was tormented with memories of each time I was short-tempered or unkind to Cody. I recited a *Hail Mary* to myself. I imagined Mary, the perfect mother, watching over Cody better than I could. I felt flawed, unworthy, and frantic. I couldn't stand feeling so restless anymore. I went into the airplane bathroom, closed my eyes and concentrated on sending a mental image to Cody, telling her to not be afraid, that God was handling everything. The moment I formed those thoughts, a crescendo of angel shivers flowed over me in waves. I was so grateful for this vivid affirmation I began to cry. Relieved, I returned to my seat and told Dennis about the angel shivers. I said with confidence, "She's okay."

When we landed in New York, I called home. Cody said she felt a little pressure around her eyes, "but I can look up, and my headache's gone."

By the time Dennis and I arrived home, Cody was cheery. "I really want Dr. Dunn to be my new neurosurgeon. She fixed my shunt without surgery. She tells me everything that's going on. I like that she doesn't just say, 'Time for a surgery.' I mean it, Mom. She's good!"

I asked Dr. Dunn if she could be Cody's doctor. She offered to discuss it with Cody's regular neurosurgeon. However, she pointed out that the shunt surgeries were always done on an emergency basis, so there was no guarantee that she'd be on call when Cody needed her.

I didn't want to offend Cody's regular doctor or compromise her care in any way. Her regular neurosurgeon wasn't a bad guy. He was actually friendly during office visits, and he treated Cody with kindness. But neither of us liked his gruff and uncommunicative manner during emergencies. That was when we didn't have a choice anyway, so no physician change was made.

Everyone in contact with Cody while we were gone reported that she handled herself with maturity in the hospital and at home. She used her support system effectively. She'd called a friend or a relative if she needed to talk. She remembered to bring up important details about her care to doctors and nurses and answered questions clearly and completely. All in all, she behaved like a mature adult.

I told her, "I am so proud of the way you managed things when we weren't here."

Cody said, "I was just taking care of myself."

Two weeks later Cody called crying from camp. "These people don't believe me, Mom. They wouldn't let me call you. My shunt isn't working, for real."

Cody had told her counselor that she was having all the symptoms of a shunt breakdown. The camp nurse saw her but was unconcerned. Cody became increasingly upset that no one took her seriously. She had finally screamed, "I could die here!"

"We're on our way, babe." I told Cody, "I want to talk to the nurse."

The nurse told me she thought my daughter was trying to manipulate us into picking her up early from camp. She added in an annoyed voice, "She's probably just homesick. And I had to call the camp doctor off the lake to speak to Cody's doctor."

I told the nurse, "Cody doesn't manipulate. *She* is the best judge of her symptoms of a shunt breakdown, which is clearly written on the summary I left with you."

The nurse didn't respond, so I said, "We'll leave now to come for Cody."

Dennis and I reached camp after dinner and found Cody in the dining hall for evening activities. Even from across the room, we saw that Cody's eyes were sunsetting. By this time, the camp doctor had also seen Cody, but he thought she was fine, perhaps tired from an overnight campout the previous evening.

Dennis scowled, "How could anyone think her eyes look normal?"

I used the camp phone to call Cody's neurosurgeon. He said to bring her straight to the emergency room. After the usual tests and a CAT scan, he wasn't entirely convinced there was a problem and decided to leave for the night. Frustrated, I asked for a neurology consult, and her neurosurgeon didn't object. The neurologist ordered an MRI. Two hours later, Cody was in surgery.

Afterwards, Cody's neurosurgeon was more communicative and forthcoming than during any previous emergency. He showed us the MRI and pointed to the end of the shunt. He explained that the top end was a quarter-inch too long. Spinal fluid drained only when it built up enough volume to push the shunt tip away from the brain matter. He'd cut off the offending quarter-inch to correct the situation. He confessed that the day of Cody's surgery was the hardest in his career. "Between Cody and another baffling case, I came close to the edge." He added, "Many of my colleagues would have gone over the edge."

I appreciated his candor and thanked him. But Cody was not happy that he shaved so much hair. She was due to have her senior picture taken a month later at the end of August.

At home Cody told me that, other than the medical emergency, she had fun at camp because she made a new friend and helped a wounded bird. "Christy thought it was neat that I'm animal rights." Cody referred to herself as "animal rights" the way a person might say "I'm French" or "I'm Presbyterian."

Cody wrote an articulate letter to the camp director, nurse, and doctor, explaining her feelings about the disrespectful treatment she experienced during her shunt emergency.

I told her, "This is an excellent letter. You express yourself very well." She muttered, "When I'm mad."

Cody had nightmares about being at camp, calling out for help and no one caring. She decided, "I won't go back to that camp. I don't feel safe there anymore."

The only response to Cody's letter came from a man not involved in the incident. His cautiously worded letter claimed that camp staff "followed appropriate procedures."

As I drove home from work a few days later, I looked up to see stunning gold columns of light with small splashes of pink spread across dark-blue slivers of clouds. I raced home to pick up Cody so she could see the beautiful cloud formations and colors. By the time we barreled toward the Lake Street Bridge to find a full view, the sky was pink. I stopped the car, and we watched the sunset. I don't recall if I pointed out to Cody that the sun was setting in the west.

I cut Cody's hair in a cute style and her senior picture turned out fine. From most angles the shorter hair around the incision wasn't noticeable. Cody began her senior year feeling good. She looked like a typical eighteen-year-old girl sitting in a wheelchair.

I didn't know it then, but Cody had entered a period of seven full years without medical emergencies of any kind.

Chapter 18

Thanks

"We can do whatever you want for Thanksgiving," I told Cody.

Dennis left for Fiji, Samoa, Tonga, and Australia for most of November and December. Since he would be gone for the greater part of the holiday season, I wanted to make our time alone more fun for Cody. She chose something we'd never do with Dennis present. We set places at the dinner table for our dogs. There was no turkey, of course, since Cody and I were both vegetarians. Before he left, Dennis had made our favorite onion quiche. Our delicious holiday meal also included peas, salad, and pumpkin pie—but the best part by far was the company.

All three dogs sat politely in chairs at the table. As soon as the meal was served, Blue leaned forward and scarfed down his food. I reminded him to sit and stay, and he did. Dan carefully put his paws on the table to reach his plate. He lapped up his dinner and sat back in the chair. But Milka sat still. Cody tried to persuade her. "It's okay, Milka. You can eat."

Milka looked pleadingly at Cody, the food, and again at Cody. A quivering two-toned whine escaped her. Cody and I burst out laughing.

Cody crooned, "Aww, Milka, honey, it's okay. Poor sweetie!"

Milka finally took a bite of quiche from a fork I held. She cautiously placed one paw on the edge of the table and leaned forward to eat. All three dogs waited patiently for dessert.

"What good manners!" Cody said. "This is the best Thanksgiving ever."

All through her senior year, Cody enjoyed the friendship of a "cute" boy named Chris. He played guitar and from time to time brought other guy friends over to see Cody. She said she liked having boys around, and she thought Chris was sweet and sensitive.

In the spring he asked Cody to the prom. She tried on a dozen dresses before choosing a black one that accentuated her ample cleavage in a tasteful way.

On prom night, our dining room was transformed into an intimate bistro. The candlelit table near the windows was surrounded by plants. Wearing tuxedo shirts and black slacks, Dennis and I served dinner to the couple as soft music played on the stereo. The hand-lettered menu read, "Welcome to the exotic kitchen of Babette and Pepi. For your dining pleasure this evening, we present a seven-course journey of culinary delight." A spoonful of lemon sorbet in a wine glass was served between courses.

Cody and Chris accepted our attentive servitude with a combination of poise and shyness. Before leaving in Chris's car, they posed for pictures in the backyard with Amy, Kari, and their dates. According to Cody, the prom itself wasn't much fun. Chris was moody and didn't even try to dance with her. They left early and rented videos. Dennis and I joined them to watch *Three Men and a Little Lady*. Cody fell asleep on the couch with her head on Chris's shoulder.

Cody was the only student in a wheelchair in South High's class of 1991. Her graduation party invitation was a collage of her school pictures from first grade through high school. Tad flew in for the ceremony and the party. Cody was proud, bright-eyed, and beautiful in her cap and gown and excitedly welcomed all her guests.

She had already received an acceptance letter from Normandale Community College. Adaptations were to be made there by the time she started classes in the fall. The administration agreed to provide an appropriate private space for Cody's bathroom needs because she had to transfer out of her chair to cath herself every few hours.

More changes were in the works when, after a brief house hunt, we found a larger home in a quiet suburb on the western edge of Minneapolis. Our little bungalow sold immediately. Dennis wasn't present for the closing or the move itself because he went to Hawaii for a week after Cody's graduation, then on to Papua New Guinea and Australia for two more weeks. Before he left, we were allowed to stack some boxes in the basement of our new house.

Cody and I continued packing and took apart beds. The roll-top desk for the computer was unwieldy. It came apart into four heavy pieces. Cody held one end of the desktop on her lap, and I lowered the other end to the floor. The two of us handled every aspect of the actual move. I couldn't have done it without her.

Even though Cody had been saying for years that she wanted a bigger house, the reality of our move was unsettling. We'd lived across the alley from the Newbergs for nine years. We loved Art, Robbie, and their five girls. On our last night in the house Robbie came over with the two youngest, Katie and Krissy. We sat in the dining room surrounded by boxes. Cody and I had been tearful off and on throughout the day. When I told Robbie how much we'd miss her, she cried, too.

By the time Dennis returned to our new house in late June, our stuff was unpacked and put away. Cody was delighted to discover that two handsome college boys lived across the street. The boys played basketball in their driveway.

"All right!" Cody said as she watched from our living room window.

Our new house needed a backyard fence for the dogs, cement walks for wheelchair access to the front and back doors, an accessible bathroom, new flooring, and a closet in Cody's room. I stipulated with the contractor we hired that I'd help with the remodel whenever I was available. I hoped my contribution would make the overall project less expensive. Dennis was now a tenured associate professor at the University with a good salary. But our new mortgage was hefty, and the remodel was pricy. With a lock box on the back door, workers came and went as needed. The project began in early July just as I left for Spain to present an art talk at the University of Madrid. I returned five days later to a house full of activity and sheetrock dust.

Cody was excited to fill me in on the goings-on while I'd been away: Dennis ran alongside her in a 5K race; she placed 33 out of 60, and fifth in the women's wheelchair division. Her name was in the paper. She showed me the number that was pinned to her T-shirt.

And, she'd met some of the neighbors. "The cute guy across the street is Joe. He plays basketball and loud music almost every day in the driveway. A lot of times he takes off his shirt. Next to them is a couple with a baby. They're both ministers in the same church."

Cody had been home for most of the construction work on her private suite, as we were now calling her bedroom, bathroom, and hall near the back door. One worker was her favorite. "You should see Ernie's butt!"

I found out right away which one was Ernie. He was the one who did all the skilled labor and directed the other workers. He wanted to show me a complication he discovered with the pipe configuration in the basement ceiling. He suggested a way to correct the problem without adding cost to the project. He explained everything to Cody as well.

Ernie found a forty-two-inch-square tub with lower-than-standard sides that Cody could easily climb into from the floor. He ensured that fixtures were within her reach and placed a holder for a handheld showerhead at a perfect height, so she could sit in the tub to take a shower or bath. He consulted her about materials and textures for flooring and walls. I often came home to find Cody chatting with Ernie while he worked.

Dennis and I both noticed that Ernie was a perfectionist. His recommendations were helpful and he found ways to save us money. He was an expert at plumbing, electricity, carpentry, roofing, and design. Dennis and I decided we didn't want anyone else working in our house except Ernie. The owner of the company was reluctant and explained that our decision would result in our project taking a lot longer because Ernie was in demand from other customers as well. I said we didn't mind.

From time to time Cody asked, "Mom, have you noticed his butt yet?"

"Aghh! I forgot again."

Cody said, "Blue acts like he's seeing his long lost friend when Ernie shows up, Mom. He gets just as excited every time. You should see how he watches Ernie."

Although I kept forgetting to notice Ernie's butt, I did notice that he was hardworking, smart, and tenderhearted. He was only thirty-seven, but his full head of wavy hair was almost entirely silver. His gentle manner and handsome appearance reminded me of Sam Elliot in movies like *Mask* or *Roadhouse*. On cigarette breaks in the backyard, Ernie tossed crabapples for

Blue to retrieve. After the third night of cleaning up crabapple vomit from the living room carpet, I asked Ernie to please not throw crabapples for Blue anymore. When I came home from work the next afternoon, Cody was sitting by the dining room window. "Look, Mom."

Ernie had cut wooden blocks with his circular saw and was throwing them for Blue. Cody and I went outside to watch. Ernie hurled a block the entire length of the yard. If Blue didn't see it land, he looked back at Ernie, who used hand gestures to direct Blue to his new toy. If Ernie waved his hand to the left and said, "Go left, left, left," Blue did. He grabbed the block and brought it back for Ernie to throw again. Blue went backward, forward, right, or left in response to the gestures and commands.

Cody hugged her dog and said, "Bluey, you are so smart!"

Dennis and I visited Normandale Community College with Cody a few times that summer. The "accessible" bathrooms did not have an appropriate surface for her to transfer onto to change her incontinent brief. Each time an alternative space was identified, we returned to see if it worked. Cody wheeled up and down the halls, read notices on the bulletin boards and checked out classrooms, labs, and auditoriums. She said, "This is a pretty cool place. I think I'll like it here."

Placement tests were given to determine Cody's first semester course choices. She worried that she wouldn't do well in English despite her success in every class Mr. Debe taught in high school. Her grades were good, and her writing was honest and entertaining. She'd written a series of inventive essays in Mr. Debe's class that began, "I woke up this morning, and I was . . . a dog, or a table." My favorite started with, "I woke up this morning, and I was a piece of dirt. I was so disgusted. I hate dirt, and there I was—a piece of it."

When a postcard came in the mail in July from CareerTrack offering a one-day seminar on grammar and punctuation, I asked Cody if she'd like to attend. She said, "I'm not too good at that stuff." We decided to go together on the Friday after Labor Day.

My parents flew to Minneapolis for Labor Day weekend. We walked around Lake of the Isles, and Dad treated us to a birthday dinner at an outdoor restaurant chosen by Cody. Although he looked thinner, Dad said he felt fine. On the last afternoon of the visit he sat on the couch with his arm around Milka, who was asleep with her snout on his leg. Cody asked, "When did you and Grandma decide to get married?"

Dad smiled and said, "When President Roosevelt raised the minimum wage from twenty-five to forty cents an hour." He talked about the early years of marriage, and Mom added details. Eventually Dad dozed off on the couch. Cody played cards with Mom at the dining room table. She'd first taught Mom how to play Uno at the anniversary celebration in Florida, but Cody had to remind her which cards to put on the pile. They both laughed as Mom mismatched colors and numbers. Suddenly Mom looked up at Cody and said, "Don't have sex until you're married!"

Cody smiled in surprise, "Don't worry, Grandma; I can't even get a date."

At the grammar and punctuation seminar in a downtown hotel, Cody and I sat at a table in the middle of the conference room. She struggled to absorb the lecture information but relaxed when we did the written exercises. We had fun deciding where to put commas, semicolons, and new-paragraph marks on the sample sheets; we looked back and forth at each other's papers.

After the class, Cody said, "That wasn't as hard as I thought."

Cody rode the Metro Mobility bus three days a week, sometimes four, and carried her schoolbooks in a backpack slung onto the handles of her wheelchair. After the first week of college she reported, "I have nice teachers in both classes."

Two weeks later she called me at work on a Friday morning, "Mom, my tire's flat and the bus is due in fifteen minutes. I've got an 11:30 class I can't miss!"

I said I'd come home right away, but I wasn't sure what I could do in time for the bus or the class. On the ten-minute drive home, I tried to recall where I'd put the bicycle pump in the new house. I didn't know of a local medical supply place, and we lived a half hour from the one we used in South Minneapolis. If I couldn't fix the tire I'd need to take her wheelchair someplace before five o'clock, or Cody would be stuck over the weekend, too. I pulled in our driveway and rushed in to find Cody sitting in a dining room chair with her elbow leaning on the kitchen table. She smiled and said, "Hi Mom."

It took a minute to absorb the scene in front of me. Cody's wheelchair was on its side on the kitchen floor next to the air compressor Ernie used for his nail guns. A damaged inner tube and some tools lay next to Cody's spare wheelchair, which had both wheels removed. A Metro Mobility driver was standing in the kitchen doorway, arms folded, with a grin on his face. Ernie was attaching a hose to the air compressor. With a loud *phsssht*, he inflated the tire.

In fluid motion, Ernie lifted the repaired wheel, snapped it onto Cody's chair, turned it upright, lifted Cody into her chair and wheeled her to the door. The Metro driver winked and took the handles to guide Cody out the back door. Cody kept smiling as she grabbed her backpack and said, "Thanks, Ernie! See ya, Mom!"

I think my mouth was still open as Ernie began to roll up the air compressor hose. I said, "That was amazing! How did you know we even had a spare wheelchair? I forgot it myself."

"I saw it one time in the garage," Ernie said as he hoisted the heavy compressor and walked toward the door.

Still overwhelmed, I put down my briefcase and helped gather some of his tools. I was so grateful, I felt like crying. I offered Ernie lunch, and we talked while we ate. He told me about his fiancée and his reservations about marriage. He wasn't sure he was ready to give up his freedom, but decided that at thirty-seven, it was time.

From previous conversations I already knew Ernie was knowledgeable about business, politics, and history. Now I learned that he was also a musician who played several instruments, including guitar and piano. He obviously loved dogs. We talked some about my animal advocacy work, writing, and, of course, Cody.

"She's a sweetheart," he said as he fed scraps of bread crust to Blue, Milka, then Dan. We talked more as he showed me how to ground an outlet.

That night, Cody said, "Ernie is my hero." *Mine, too*, I thought.

When Ernie came the following week, Cody presented him with a navy-blue Normandale sweatshirt and a thank-you note. She told me, "Ernie went to Normandale, too."

After he left that day, Cody said, "Blue and Ernie love each other so much, Mom. Blue gets more excited seeing Ernie than he gets about anything, and he stays near Ernie all day. I've been thinking that maybe Blue should be Ernie's dog. I think he'd be happier with Ernie."

I saw that Cody was sincere. "You'd give up your dog for Ernie?"

Cody said, "I love Blue, and I don't want to give him up. But if he'd be happier with Ernie, it might be the right thing to do. Ernie loves him."

"That's really sweet and unselfish, babe. He does love Blue. But Ernie works long days and lives more than an hour away from here. You found Blue, and he loves you, too. Besides, now that Ernie is our friend, Blue will always be able to see him."

Cody scratched Blue's ears and said, "They sure love each other."

Chapter 19

Individuation

CODY CAME HOME from a class in November just as Ernie finished a project in our guest room. The three of us chatted over a cup of tea. Cody's phone rang and she said, "It's only Sharon. I'll call her back."

Ernie looked at her quickly and said, "Never take your friends for granted." Cody said okay and went to her room to call Sharon back. While she was gone Ernie commented, "I think Cody's depressed about school."

I asked, "Why do you think that? She's getting good grades so far."

"I don't think it's the academic part. It's the social aspects. She wants to fit in, have dates, and she's not as mature as the people around her. There are probably some not-so-nice kids at Normandale, too. I remember some snotty kids there who picked on shy kids."

Ernie's observation sounded logical, but I had not noticed Cody feeling down. I told him, "She wants her own apartment. Independence has been the goal all along. We're looking into the logistics and the services available. But I worry whether she's emotionally ready to live on her own."

He said, "She does lack anecdotal contributions to conversations— her own stories."

Ernie's words sounded familiar. My friend Shelley had recently said she noticed Cody's silence during group interactions. She'd say, "Mom, tell that story . . ." and I'd say, "You tell the story." Cody would answer, "But you tell it better."

I asked Ernie, "What could help her with that?"

"Have you ever gone away and left her on her own?"

"Not really. She always has someone stay with her."

"Maybe you and Dennis could go away for a night. See how she feels being completely on her own. It might build her confidence."

That evening while Cody scooped out the dogs' dinner, I told her some of what Ernie had said. I asked, "Are you depressed about the social aspect of school?"

"I don't think so," Cody answered thoughtfully. "I really worry more about the academic part. I always think I can't do it."

"But you are doing it. You're maintaining a high B average."

"Yeah, I guess so." Cody went to her room to finish her homework.

I was drawing at the table when she wheeled back into the kitchen and said, "I've been thinking about what Ernie said. He might be right. The academic part is fine. I love college, especially Willie's class."

"Are you depressed that you're not more active socially? That you aren't dating?"

Cody shrugged and said, "Yeah, but everybody feels that way. Everybody gets depressed from time to time."

"You're so wise. I love you," I told her. "Maybe you need more autonomy, especially from me. Maybe you need to do more things that have *nothing* to do with me, *or* Dennis. So many personal things related to your disability have sort of forced you to depend on us more than most non-disabled people your age might. I don't want to be one of those clingy mothers who prevents my kid from being strong on her own. I need to let go of you in more ways."

Cody thought that made sense. We talked about our changing roles now that she was a young adult of nineteen. She had cried only recently saying, "Your best friend is Shelley, but my best friend is you." I had answered, "Honey, you always have me. You need lots of other best friends."

Now Cody said, "Okay, then let's look at apartments!"

"Okay, and you let me know if I treat you like a kid. I won't remind you about chores or homework anymore."

"You'll still help me if I need it though, right?"

"Sure, but I'll wait until you ask."

"Okay then." Cody looked over my shoulder while I sketched with oil pastels and said, "If I could paint like you, I'd do it to show off all the time."

I countered, "You *do* paint well. You're a good artist. You've been in the Sister Kenny shows every year. That bird you drew was terrific!"

Cody said, "I decided I don't want to be an artist. I'm not going to be in the Sister Kenny show anymore."

Without showing my surprise, I asked, "Why not?"

"It's hard work. I don't want to have to work that hard at it."

"It is work," I admitted. "You're right about that."

On the phone later with Shelley, I described the conversation with Cody. Shelley was a psychiatric social worker, generous with her observations on human behavior. She said, "Cody is individuating." We talked more about behavioral concepts like emancipation and enmeshment. Shelley observed, "It's too easy for your opinions to become Cody's opinions."

I remembered Cody as a child asking, "Are we Democrats?" I knew whatever I answered would become her view. I encouraged her to decide those things for herself.

I told Shelley, "I feel guilty pushing her away."

"You're too hard on yourself," Shelley insisted. "It's normal. Cody needs to emancipate. Mother birds push their babies out of the nest."

The night after Thanksgiving, I heard Cody crying in her room. I went in to ask her what was wrong. She held Milka and sobbed, "I had a bad dream that Grandpa and Milka both died." My father was home from the hospital after prostate surgery and was undergoing daily radiation treatment. I assured Cody, "He said he felt okay when we talked on the phone yesterday."

"But my dreams always come true!" she cried.

I hugged her. "I'm sorry, sweetie. We'll call in the morning and check again. On the bright side, Richard comes tomorrow."

The "little brother" Cody never had, as she once called my younger brother Richard, arrived the next day. His visit cheered up Cody quite a bit. We laughed hard at dinner as Richard and I shared stories about being Cody's age. I forgot she was listening and said a few things that widened her eyes. "Mu-u-ther!" she grinned, raising her eyebrows. We laughed. I said, "I'm lucky to have a perfect daughter, and not the rabble-rouser our poor mother had!"

Starting the day after Christmas, Cody stayed at her friend Sharon's apartment for a week to take care of her cat while Sharon visited family in North Dakota for Chanukah. Cody called home after the first night to report that she was fine. She sounded excited. "I was too nervous to eat yesterday. I went to bed at midnight and woke up at 4:45."

She went out during the day and called me at work a few times for various things. In the evening, she visited with Sharon's upstairs neighbor and called Dennis and me later to say goodnight. Her friend Yolanda from Normandale came for dinner the third night. Cody took a bus home in the middle of the day to take a bath in her own tub and pick up groceries. While she was home I made a date with her to see a movie on Sunday.

I was beginning to be able to imagine Cody living on her own and our making plans like these. It felt nice. Dennis and I both missed Cody that week. But it was fun missing her, knowing she was doing something that made her feel powerful and independent. With Cody gone, all three dogs piled onto our bed at night. Dennis didn't appreciate that as much as I did.

Our water heater sprung a leak on New Year's Eve day. I called Ernie. "It's no rush; it's a slow leak. I put a bowl under it. But I wanted to thank you for your excellent advice about Cody."

He asked, "How's she doing at Sharon's?" I told him how Cody took a bus to buy groceries, hosted a dinner and visited people.

"This'll build her self-confidence. Something similar made a difference to me at her age."

Agreeing, I said, "I feel bad that I didn't see how important it was."

Ernie said, "Sometimes it takes someone from the outside."

At 12:07 a.m., January 1, Cody called to say, "Happy New Year!"

She came home the following day just as Dennis left for New Orleans. Her recent melancholy was gone. She exuded a striking new confidence. She came to my room that night to tell me about a boy she liked at Normandale. As she said a quick goodnight and went off with the dogs to bed, I started to think maybe Cody wasn't the one with a problem separating from me. Maybe I was the one having trouble. With that, and problems Dennis and I were having again, I decided to make an appointment for a tune-up with our marriage counselor.

Cody became a Lutheran in March. The pastors next door to the handsome neighbor boys had invited her to their church. After attending the Lutheran church for several Sundays, she invited Dennis and me to come with her. People greeted Cody by name as we entered the church and she introduced us to folks.

Though Dennis no longer wanted to move to Australia, he was now considering a job offer from a university in St. Louis. He said it would be a good career move "if the money's right." Cody and I had the same reaction; neither of us wanted to move again. Dennis wasn't sure he did either, but he made another trip to St. Louis to learn more about the opportunity. I checked into services there for those with disabilities and found no public transportation options for people in wheelchairs. After further discussion Dennis decided not to take the offer.

The very next day, Cody gave me an urgent message as I walked in the door after work. "Uncle Charlie called. Grandpa's in the hospital!"

I called immediately and spoke to Dad. In a lot of pain that afternoon, he had driven straight from work to the hospital. But he was going home in the morning. A different tone in Dad's voice prompted me to ask him if I could call his doctor. The oncologist returned my call immediately. I told him, "My father sounds like he thinks he's dying."

The doctor said, "He is. Cancer has spread to his bones and internal organs. He's deteriorating."

My mind raced. "All my brothers and I live in different states. We need to make plans. What is your best guess on how long he has left?"

"I'd say three weeks."

I thought doctors didn't give such specific predictions, but I was grateful this one did. My brothers and I worked as a team to help our parents in overlapping shifts in Pittsburgh over the next weeks. Everyone in the family advised against Cody going, but she said, "I want to see Grandpa, too." She had second thoughts when she spoke to Dad by phone. He sounded weak and breathless and had trouble talking. Cody cried each morning and night for her Grandpa.

I told her, "It's your decision, babe. You can come for a couple days while I'm there, if you want. If you decide not to go, that's okay, too."

I spent five days with my father. He was in pain much of the time.

Dennis and Cody called the first morning for an update. I said, "We were up before dawn. Dad takes tons of pills at all different times. I already took Billy and Richard to the airport. A hospice nurse comes at 3:30, and Dad wants me to teach Mom how to drive, pay bills, and get cash from ATMs. It's not even noon, and I'm wiped."

Cody asked, "How's Grandma?"

"She's a nervous wreck. This whole thing is freaking her out. She wants to help Dad. She keeps telling him to eat. He only ate one bite of an avocado at breakfast."

"Get Grandpa a balloon from me that says *I love you* on it, okay, Mom?"

Dad cried when I gave him the balloon from Cody. He cried again telling Mom how he'd be torn up if she got cancer like Joe Clark's wife, Betty, did after Joe died. He insisted I take Mom for a mammogram right away and made me promise to be sure she'd have regular check-ups. I'd never seen my father cry, but he cried frequently in our last five days together. Every four hours, I rubbed his back and Mom massaged his feet until his pain medication took effect. Then we talked and laughed about cancer, death, philosophy, and family.

"I don't know how I am going to get everything done by Sunday night," I told Cody and Dennis on Friday.

Cody offered, "I'll help. My flight gets in tomorrow night. I don't think you should tell Grandpa I'm coming. He might worry that I'm flying alone." Mom and I took Cody's suggestion and didn't mention her plans to Dad.

Late Friday afternoon Dad was moaning. His pain medication wasn't working and he described a new symptom. He said it felt like razors were cutting him when he tried to pee. A dozen phone calls later, Dad had new prescriptions from two different sources. I rubbed his back as he leaned forward on the kitchen table. He said, "You're a good girl. I'm amazed by what you accomplished with doctors, nurses, and pharmacies after 4:30 on a Friday. I figured I'd be miserable all weekend."

"It's from years of advocating for Cody. No never means no; it just means try something different."

Cody cancelled her flight Saturday morning. She explained, "It was a tough decision. I kept thinking: shall I stay here, or go there and risk scaring myself?" She spoke with Dad by phone, and he agreed she made the right choice.

Dad's doctor's estimate was off only by a day. Cody and Dennis stayed home when I returned to Pittsburgh for my father's funeral. I stayed an extra week and, at Mom's request, slept in Dad's bed. Cody called several times each day, and we talked and talked. I felt her neediness and her loss, but was unable to give her much. I felt empty and tired.

Dennis had gone to Denver the morning I flew home. I took a cab from the airport. Cody and I went to Burger King that night for veggie Whoppers and more talk about her grandfather.

Chapter 20

Change

THE PHONE RANG. Cody said, "It's probably Ernie saying his nose broke, or his eye fell out." Ernie promised many times to work on the house, only to later cancel.

Dennis commented, "I feel like I'm in a *Murphy Brown* episode."

Murphy Brown's house painter was a permanent fixture, like a member of the family. Ernie was like that TV character with us. Dennis and I hired him for every project and repair. But his boss kept sending him on other jobs, or else he was sick. We'd see him for a few days, then not again for another week or so.

My brush was dipped, and I'd begun to paint one evening in early June when Cody said she wanted to tell me something.

"Sharon asked me if you and Ernie are having an affair."

By now I considered Ernie a best friend. I adored him and didn't hide my affection. He had commented, "I'm gonna hurt myself when I fall off *this* pedestal." However, despite my attraction to him, I had no illicit intentions. I had a fantasy at the time that he and I could be like Olympic skaters Torvill and Dean—an intimate working relationship between two people married to others. I asked Cody, "Why does Sharon think that?"

"When she was here the other day it was quiet while you and Ernie worked."

"We were working on the closet doors. Nothing sexy about it." I explained further, "No one questions Dennis having women friends. He socializes with female students and wives of his friends. His running partner is a woman; he's friends with most of his old girlfriends, and he's staying alone with Shelley right now in Phoenix."

"That's true," Cody agreed.

I continued, "When I took dance lessons with David, Lyn thought he was my boyfriend. When I walked around the lake every week with Father Tom, someone could have thought we were having an affair. People just think things."

Cody lowered her eyes. "I told Dad I was concerned that your friendship with Ernie could threaten your marriage."

Dennis and I were having problems again, but I tried not to discuss that with Cody unless she mentioned it. She added, "But Dad told me you'd never break up because of Ernie."

"He's right, sweetie. I adore Ernie. You, Dennis, Sharon—*every*body knows that. You adore him, too. But you also know the problems Dennis and I've had. If we ever break up, it won't be because of another person."

Cody spent ten days in July at a camp in northern Minnesota for young adults with disabilities. When Dennis and I drove there to bring her home, she introduced us to a counselor she befriended. On the ride home she told us that he was hearing-impaired and he'd been her date for the dance on the final night. She smiled. "I had a great time but I'm glad to go home to rest. I forgot my headphones and I didn't get much alone time. I realized again at camp that I like a lot of quiet time." She told me more camp stories while I was in the bathtub that evening.

Dennis was leaving at the end of July for a month in Australia. Ernie had agreed to take time off from his regular job to replace our roof, and I would help. Dennis asked us to do the job while he was gone so he'd miss the noise and mess. Since the roof had a gentle pitch, Ernie was confident the two of us could do it within a week.

Cody and I took Dennis to the airport and spent the next nine days renting videos, shopping, and going to movies. Then I had a long talk with Cody. I told her Dennis and I needed time apart, that I'd probably move out of the house when he returned from Oz. Cody had a worried look as I explained that this change was not intended to be permanent, but it was necessary, and it had nothing to do with her. I reminded her that she was on a waiting list for an accessible apartment; it wouldn't be long before she'd have her own place. I promised, "We'll visit each other and go places all the time, just like we do now."

We continued to discuss her fears daily. Cody said she was afraid of losing the material and emotional support that Dennis and I gave her. Those weren't her exact words, but that was the gist of her concern. I told her, "You will never, ever, *ever* lose me. As long as I live and breathe, I'm here for you, babe. You are the most important person in the world to me. You won't lose me no matter what. And Dennis loves you; that won't change, either."

Dennis was due home a few days before Cody turned twenty, so her usual birthday planning was knocked askew by this development. She decided not to have a party. Tad flew in for a four-day visit, but we didn't mention the coming change to him. Cody asked us to sing the songs we used to sing at bedtime when she was little. Tad's visit was so comfortable and fun that Cody asked, "Why didn't *we* stay a family?" Before Tad or I could answer, she said, "Never mind. I know. I know."

Cody's mood alternated between sad, tense, and mad. I hated being a source of her anxiety. I told her I was very sorry. "It's okay if you're mad at me. But I hope you don't stay mad too long. I love you."

Watching Dennis on a TV news interview about his demographic research on the American family, Cody said, "He looks unhappy, Mom."

After two weeks of rain in early August, Ernie and I finally got together to begin work on the roof. Cody was experimenting with a recipe in the kitchen when we stopped work after our second day in the hot sun. Ernie came inside for a cold drink before heading home. Cody listened as we discussed a problem we encountered with the roof. The shingles were double-nailed. Ernie said, "There's no way we can finish in a week without help." Ernie and I were due back at our jobs the following week. Neither of us knew anyone who could help us on such short notice.

Cody's eyes lit up as she suggested, "Maybe Mr. Debe can help. He does summer jobs."

She made the call. Mr. Debe had a back injury; however, he knew a painting crew that was available. Ernie and I bought more roofing shovels, and three Irish college students helped tear off the old roof. They were hard workers who rarely took breaks despite the heat. Cody brought them cold drinks. They talked with her and played catch with Blue.

Cody took calls from Mom and my brother Richard that week. When she told them I was up on the roof, they both asked the same question in the same way. "Ernie's up there with her; isn't he?" When Cody answered yes, each had said in relief, "Oh, good."

Cody laughed telling Ernie, "Grandma and Uncle Richard both have more faith in a person they've never met than in Mom's ability to get off the roof!"

As the dumpster company hauled away the refuse from the roof, Ernie thanked Cody again. "We couldn't have done this without you, Cody. Your idea to call Mr. Debe made all the difference."

She lowered her chin in an aww-shucks smile.

The Saturday night before Dennis returned home, Cody went alone to the wedding of the older of the two handsome brothers she'd watched play basketball from her window. She came home late, full of chatter. "I had fun, and I danced."

Upon his return, Dennis helped me find an apartment close to the hospital where I worked. He co-signed the lease and helped me shop for extra furnishings. Cody watched his moods to make sure he hadn't changed toward her. Rather than involve her in conversations about our separation, Dennis and I each suggested that she talk about her concerns with Bob, her Lutheran pastor across the street. She said Bob was sympathetic and supportive.

The first week after I moved out was the hardest on Cody. On my first night in the apartment, she and I talked on the phone until we fell asleep. The next day Dennis and I took Cody to a Color Me Bad concert at the Minnesota State Fair for her birthday. Cody smiled, clapped, and danced in her chair.

Our usual practice was to leave big concerts before the encore song to avoid being stuck in the middle of a crowd. As this encore began, Cody dashed ahead toward the exit, wheeling past others in the front row. She was surprised and elated to notice Janet Jackson sitting a few seats away. A tall burly man tried to stop Cody by grabbing her wheelchair handles. She thrust ahead assertively, and Jackson's bodyguard let go. Cody smiled a hello as she whizzed past Janet Jackson. She was thrilled that Jackson smiled and waved back.

On the first Sunday in my apartment I invited Cody and Dennis for dinner. Knowing my limited cooking skills, Dennis offered to bring the food. We had a pleasant meal. Dennis left early to go to a movie with friends, and Cody stayed for the evening.

We compared notes in the coming days. Cody and I both noticed that planning ahead to see each other was fun and made us appreciate our time together more.

As it became more obvious to Dennis and me that we were moving rapidly toward the decision to divorce, Cody maintained a sardonic sense of humor when the three of us were together. During dinner after two weeks apart, Cody asked about a movie date Dennis and I had. After we each presented our assessments of the date, Cody said, "You are *both* pitiful."

After three weeks, Cody told me, "You and Dad are so different, and I'm different with each of you. But I miss seeing your friends. I like your friends."

At six weeks, Cody said, "You and Dad are definitely better off apart."

When I stayed with Cody and the dogs for several days while Dennis was away, Cody told me, "I want to move out as soon as possible. I'd rather live on my own than with either parent. My insecure side wants the family together, but I'm ready to move on."

I said, "Okay, let's check on the waiting lists for accessible apartments. They said it might be two years, but you never know. Things change all the time."

That weekend, Cody and I helped our friend Roberta with some political campaigning. She was running for state senator from her district. She walked with crutches due to partial paralysis in her legs from post-polio syndrome. Her campaign focused on healthcare for the disabled. This was an issue that our senator, Paul Wellstone, and his wife, Sheila, supported wholeheartedly. They'd offered to spend a day door-knocking for Roberta's campaign.

Wind blew continuously on the sunny October day. Cody and I enjoyed every minute. The Wellstones were warm and informal with us. We all talked and laughed with Roberta as we rushed from house to house in a West Bloomington neighborhood, passing out flyers and talking to residents. I pushed Cody's wheelchair up the hills. Roberta moved more slowly on her crutches. Cody cheered her on with a smile. "Go get 'em!"

By the end of the day we were all tired—in a good way. Roberta thanked everyone for the help and told Cody, "I really appreciated your enthusiasm. You're a loyal campaigner!"

That night Cody and I went to a Kathy Mattea concert at the Guthrie Theater. We harmonized to her songs on the drive home and collapsed into bed.

Cody was maintaining an A in English, but worried about failing her health class. Despite interest in the subject and fondness for the teacher, she hated the class. I helped her by reading the textbook out loud; then we discussed the topics.

I found a completed questionnaire in a pile of her school papers wherein Cody listed her highest priorities in life as "independence" and "helping others." For qualities she most liked about herself, she wrote, "I'm nice to people, sweet, nice to animals, and I can deal with things." I felt so good reading that last one.

She had written several one-page versions of her autobiography. One began, "I will start by writing about my feelings when people who are full-blooded white American citizens without physical problems discriminate against people who don't fit that description."

Cody met with an astrologer that month who told her, "You're a healer, artist, teacher, therapist, and lover of life. You are an authentic inspiration to many people, and you always will be."

That description sounded on the mark to me. I thought of Cody as a healer. Whenever I felt sick, I thought her prayers were the ones that made the difference.

Ernie called in early November to tell me he'd broken up with the woman he'd once planned to marry. He was now living with a friend in St. Paul. He said it was a tough break-up and I probably wouldn't hear from him for a while. He asked how Cody was doing. He hadn't seen her in more than two months. I told him, "She asks about you, too."

"Tell her I'll call her soon; we'll meet for lunch at Normandale."

After I hung up with Ernie, the phone rang again right away. Cody said, "I just called to get some sympathy. I have a migraine."

A fellow migraine-sufferer, I was able to give her lots of sympathy. I asked, "Did you try Mom's reflexology technique?"

My mother taught Cody which points to press on the hand to relieve colds or headaches. When I had a migraine, Cody squeezed hard on a spot on the webbed area of my palm between the thumb and forefinger. Piercing pain in my hand usually took my mind off the headache. I reacted by crossing my eyes and scrunching up my face as Cody squeezed, and she laughed uproariously. The method actually worked, sometimes.

Cody said, "Good idea. I'll try that."

"Ernie just called and asked about you. He wants to meet you for lunch at school."

"Cool."

Cody and I flew to Pittsburgh for Thanksgiving. She wanted to make sure her grandmother was okay on the first big holiday since my father's death.

The doorways in Mom's house were too narrow for Cody's latest wheelchair. I had to take the bedroom door off its hinges. Cody had to rely on my help when she cathed herself or changed clothes. She had not depended on anyone else for assistance with such personal care in quite some time, and she was not comfortable doing so now. She had gained fifteen pounds in recent months; I couldn't lift her anymore. We tried to figure out how to raise her from the floor to her chair. I lay face down and she climbed on my back. I tried to rise up on my hands and knees, but I fell sideways. We rolled over laughing. What finally worked was when Cody put her forearms on the bed or couch and I lifted her by the ankles, guiding her forward like a wheelbarrow onto the surface.

Aside from those challenges, the visit was stress-free. Mom was doing well and had new friendships with other women who lost husbands. My brother Richard, his wife, and daughter were there, too. Five-year-old Joanna climbed onto Cody's lap and they wheeled around the house, played games together and drew pictures. Cody said, "I just *love* my sweet little cousin."

Christmas was the next milestone with Cody since my move to an apartment. I invited her to spend Christmas Eve overnight with me. Dennis dropped her off. We opened presents for each other and listened to music. I invited my friend David to dinner to make the holiday more festive. He was a psychologist who was charming and funny; whenever I saw him, we talked late into the night. He brought presents for Cody and me. Her eyes sparkled as they talked and she laughed comfortably with him until after midnight, sharing stories about her surgeries, health scares, and adventures. When David left, Cody said, "He's so cute; I had to try hard not to just stare at him."

Days later Cody confessed that she'd been "gossiping" with Tad when he called on Christmas night. They had discussed which man, David or Ernie, would be the best new husband for me! My divorce from Dennis was not yet final, hardly the time for me to be thinking about another husband. However, I was already sure about one thing: I was in love with Ernie.

Starting that weekend, Ernie, Cody, and I went places together once or twice a week. Like my mother, Cody was a shrewd observer of people. If she ever warned me about a person's motives, she was proven right every time. Mom once said that Cody had the "gift of discernment."

After an evening at a country western bar, watching people dance the two-step, Cody told me, "I had a chance to study Ernie tonight while you two were talking. He looks all macho, but he's softhearted. I think he really loves you. But I'm not sure he's ready to be tied down in a new relationship." I appreciated that my daughter was looking out for me.

I was feeling pretty good about how much and how well Cody was doing independently. She joined an adaptive hockey team and took art classes at Courage Center. I drove her there if she couldn't get a Metro ride.

Every week or so she rode a bus downtown to visit an elderly woman from St. Albert's who now lived in a nursing home.

Cody was already responsible for the care and feeding of the dogs, but now she also took care of the house when Dennis was away for long stretches. One thing she couldn't do was the laundry because the washer and dryer were in the basement. When Dennis left near the end of January for a month in Australia, I did her laundry and we played Scrabble and I told her how impressed I was with her ability to take care of herself. To Cody, the most exciting symbol of her autonomy was having her own credit card.

In February, Ernie and his piano moved into my apartment. Cody invited us to a Valentine's party she and Sharon hosted in Sharon's building. Ernie and I picked up refreshments, blew up balloons, and stayed for the start of the party. When we came back later to help clean up, Cody was happy with her party's success. "My friends said you're so pretty, Mom. A couple of them told me they liked my dad, too. They thought Ernie was my dad. I didn't correct them. I'd like him to be my dad. It would be just like *Three Men and a Baby*."

At one of her weekly hockey games, Cody mentioned that players on her team usually went to a bar after the game. She couldn't go along because she didn't have a ride. "Besides, the other players are like a clique; they don't include me."

When Ernie heard that, he said, "Then we'll all go after the game." Cody smiled. "Cool!"

At the bar we ordered food and drinks, listened to the music, and played darts. Ernie put his arm around Cody when they talked. I saw in her face how much she enjoyed the way he treated her. When we took her home, he kissed her cheek and she didn't scrunch up her shoulder like she did with most people. My feelings for Ernie swelled beyond previous limits, seeing how consistently natural, protective, and kind he was to Cody.

In March, Cody invited Ernie and me to a concert. Pierce, her old babysitter from Philadelphia, was in a new band. He was appearing at First Avenue, the nightclub where Prince filmed *Purple Rain*. The music was loud, mostly hard rock with blues mixed in. Pierce gave a public "shout out" to Cody in the audience. This was the first of many times Cody went to places where Pierce played. She was his loyal fan, and they exchanged letters between gigs.

The week after Easter, Cody was informed that she was at the top of the waiting list for an apartment. The building was still under construction in Hopkins exactly five miles west of Dennis's house. She could move into her own place by the end of the year. Her excitement was uncontained. She clipped Sunday ads for furniture and spent a large portion of her savings on a sofabed so friends could stay overnight at her apartment. She transferred on and off the couch in the outlet store to make sure it was the perfect firmness. Cody created her own temporary living room in Dennis's spare bedroom. Her second purchase was a recliner. She secured her wheelchair brakes, rolled onto the chair, leaned back and said, "Ahh, nice."

When Ernie and I came home after midnight on a Saturday in April, the phone answering machine was blinking; the message was heartbreaking. Cody cried, "Mom! Milka died."

Cody had returned from an evening with friends to find Blue barking in alarm. He led her to Milka, who lay as though asleep on the living room carpet. Blue ran, barking, in frantic circles around Milka. When Cody couldn't reach me, she called the neighbors. The pastors came right away, wrapped Milka in a blanket and laid her in the garage. After they left, Cody cried and hugged Blue and Dan. Dennis arrived home around the same time I heard the message. He would bury Milka under a bush in the backyard the next day. But that night my girl had been alone, and I could hear the break in her heart at the loss of her "little mother."

Milka was fifteen when she died. She'd been part of our family all the years Dennis and I were married. We'd adopted her within weeks of our wedding; our divorce had become final only weeks before she died.

Chapter 21

Moving

CODY HAD NEWS in June. She'd been applying for summer jobs and proudly announced that Computer City hired her as a greeter. Ernie and I visited the store a few days into her new employment. Cody wore a yellow employee shirt and cheerfully welcomed shoppers. She found the work profoundly boring but stuck with it even though her hours changed daily. Metro Mobility didn't provide or change rides on short notice or pick up after nine at night. Despite Cody's request for a set work schedule, last-minute changes continued and she was forced to resign.

Julie, the mother of the handsome boys across the street, offered Cody a summer job as a clerical aide at an insurance firm. Cody said, "It's a *real* job. I have to dress for business."

I said, "That's great! Let's go out and buy some new clothes."

A few weeks later Julie told me that Cody was an able and professional addition to the office. Cody reported, "This is the best job I've ever had."

Ernie and I had news for Cody, too. "We bought a small house with big potential. And it's only eight blocks from you. You are invited for lunch on Sunday and Ernie's family will be there, too."

Cody was immediately drawn to Ernie's mother. Lorraine was soft-spoken and sweet, and a bit frail from a recent fall. While Ernie's aunt, brother, sister, and their families played games in our yard, Cody talked with Lorraine. Cody said she wanted to come over from now on whenever Lorraine visited.

Ernie and I had begun a major renovation when Cody brought Dennis to see our house one summer afternoon. The porch was torn off and some walls were removed. Dennis tilted back Cody's wheelchair to lift her through a temporary front door. Cody had arranged the visit for a specific purpose. Dennis hadn't seen Ernie in the past year, and she wanted to be sure there was no awkwardness between them. "I'll be twenty-one in six weeks, and I want us all together for my birthday."

Dennis and Ernie cheerfully agreed to her idea.

Cody changed the subject as she held up her hand. "Look, Mom. This happens lately whenever I touch anything cold. It feels like an itchy burn." Her hand had a rash and puffiness where she had touched her glass of ice-cold lemonade.

With a neurologist the following week, Cody was asked to describe the problem. She said, "Give me some ice and I'll show you." The doctor filled a cup of crushed ice from a machine in the hall, and Cody put a small chunk on her forearm. Every part of her skin touched by the ice or the melting drops turned bright red and formed a burn welt. The doctor's eyes widened watching the skin react so quickly. Cody asked, "Do you want me to do it again?"

"No!" the doctor said firmly, "Don't *ever* do that again!"

The neurologist called the allergy "cold urticaria" and advised Cody to avoid touching anything cold. A tall order for anyone living in Minnesota! She was scheduled for a follow-up CAT scan to be sure nothing else was wrong. Nothing was. This was just a new item to add to Cody's medical summary.

Lewis called Cody a couple of weeks before her birthday and said, "Orlando and I decided to call our old girlfriends." Cody had stopped thinking of Lewis as a "boyfriend" by the end of high school. She'd commented at the time, "We're just friends. He's not ready for a *mature* relationship." They'd not seen each other since graduation. Now Cody heard Lewis acknowledge for the first time that he had actually thought of Cody as a girlfriend. She invited him to her birthday party.

The phone rang at 6:08 on the morning of August 27 and a rascally voice asked, "Remember what you were doing twenty-one years ago this *exact* minute?"

"Happy birthday, sweetie."

Cody giggled. "I thought I'd wake you up again like I did back then."

I laughed. "I love you, babe. I'll see you tonight."

Dennis hosted a party for Cody that night. The house looked wonderful. Dennis had decorated with balloons and streamers and prepared lots of food. When Ernie and I arrived, Blue ran to Ernie and shook with excitement; Dan jumped into my arms. Friends in wheelchairs were eating at the dining-room table. Others sat around the living room with plates of food. There were family friends, friends from St. Albert's, from high school, the pastors from across the street and, of course, the Debes. Cody was surrounded by people she loved.

She continued to celebrate the following night in a downtown hotel room with a couple of girlfriends. Lewis, Orlando, Dennis, Ernie, and I joined the girls for pizza. Ernie and I had arranged for a singing telegram. A handsome young man with a boom box sang to Cody as he tore off his clothes. The singing stripper wiggled and danced for her, wearing nothing but a brief thong covering his "privates." Cody laughed so hard that I thought she'd throw up. Her face flushed as she gasped in laughter.

Ernie leaned close to her and asked, "Are you all right?"

With a smile Cody panted, "Oh, yeah!"

She laughed the hardest when she noticed Orlando and Lewis trying to move as far away as possible from the gyrating stripper.

Kathy Mattea was back at the Guthrie Theater in October. Ernie went with Cody this time. I overheard her tell a friend, "Mom's boyfriend is cool. Sometimes he goes out just with me. I'm really the one who noticed him first. I won't say what body part I noticed first—now that he's like a father to me."

The day after the concert Cody was excited by news that she could move into her own apartment in December. Dennis wanted the dogs moved out at the same time. So Ernie and I built a fence for our yard so Blue and Dan could live with us when the time came. Now that having her own place was almost a reality, Cody said moving away from home was "a little scary." She added, "Blue looked upset when he saw me packing."

Cody was given first choice of space in her new building. The one-bedroom apartments were all the same, with a combination kitchen/living room and large bathroom with wheel-in shower. The building had three floors and an elevator. Cody decided she'd feel safest on the main floor. She didn't want to risk being stranded on an upper floor if a power failure occurred. She chose the unit next to the front entrance so she could watch comings and goings from her windows and feel close to other people. She'd be able to see the Metro Mobility bus when it came to pick her up.

Ernie and I bought her a bed with built-in drawers underneath. Removing the casters made it the right height for Cody to easily climb from the floor onto the bed, and from the bed to her wheelchair. She'd already spent most of her savings but still needed curtains, a kitchen table, utensils and dishes, bathroom supplies, lamps, and bedding. We had a talk about money, the importance of paying bills on time, and not overspending on her credit card.

The state government provided Cody with medical insurance coverage and a few hundred dollars a month. To be eligible for this benefit she was required to fill out multiple-paged forms and provide copies of several types of verification that confirmed her disability status and finances. Cody and I worked on the project together. Reaching anyone by phone for advice or direction was difficult. Cody and I took turns listening to a recording that repeated the same message for thirty minutes before a real person answered the phone.

"This is complicated!" Cody observed.

I agreed. "I don't know how some people can do this. It's a lot to figure out." And we didn't yet know that the extensive application process had to be redone in its entirety every year.

Because Cody's apartment building was created as subsidized housing for people with disabilities, rent was calculated to be about a quarter of her Social Security disability income. Cody opened a checking account at a local bank. After paying rent and utility bills, remaining dollars could be used for groceries, clothes, household supplies, and entertainment. If she was very careful with her money, she could buy something inexpensive for her apartment every month or so.

On the second Sunday in December, Cody slept in her new apartment for the first time. She and I talked on the phone in bed that night and compared notes on the adjustment.

She asked, "How are the dogs?"

"Dan's asleep on my side of the bed; Blue can't get close enough to Ernie."

Cody said, "Awww, that's so sweet."

One week later, Cody hosted a housewarming party. Ernie and I brought extra folding chairs and helped set up snacks and drinks. Fresh flowers sat in a vase on the kitchen table. One of my paintings was centered over the couch. Another hung above a bookcase. The television and VCR were stacked on the right side of her desk in the corner. Her recliner divided the living room space from the kitchen.

Cody shouted, "The family's here!" and showed Ernie's family her bedroom with its new bedspread and her bathroom with large wheel-in shower. The living room/kitchen was soon lined with guests holding paper plates with cookies, chips, and dip. Everyone adjusted positions when anyone arrived in a wheelchair. Cody sat among her guests, talking and laughing. She opened a few gifts: colorful cloth napkins and matching placemats, a tablecloth, candles, and dishtowels. Dennis brought a colorful serving tray. As guests left, Cody thanked everyone for coming and said, "Please stop by any time."

Ernie and I stayed to help her clean up and put away folding chairs. With a satisfied grin, Cody said, "That was great. I love parties."

Cody called me at work or at home several times a day as she settled into her new routines. She started most calls with, "I just called to say hello." If there was a problem or she needed something, she began, "Mom, this is important!" In the evenings, we talked on the phone at least once while watching TV or lying in bed.

After a few days, I stopped by with new bath towels. A welcome mat lay inside her door. The apartment was tidy, her bed was made, and the kitchen was clean. Cody graciously invited me to stay for a dinner of cheese sandwiches.

As she met other residents in her building, Cody saw that many didn't have family who could provide the extras she had. She told me, "I feel guilty having such a nice place. I have much more than a lot of my friends."

She remained sensitive to these discrepancies and often gave away her things to others.

Cody was eligible for help from a personal care attendant on a daily basis. The county, home-care agencies and clients referred to these caregivers as PCAs. The range of help provided was related to personal body care and assistance with grocery shopping, meal preparation, and light housekeeping. The county called these "activities of daily living." This benefit required another yearly evaluation and application process that included an assessment by a county nurse who determined the number of hours Cody was eligible to receive.

The nurse made an appointment to see Cody's apartment and conduct the interview. I was glad I was there for the conversation; the meeting was difficult for Cody. She had struggled since childhood to do things for herself, and I'd always supported her healthy desire for self-sufficiency. As she answered the nurse's questions, Cody had trouble admitting that she needed help with anything. I felt sorry to have to point out to the nurse, and to Cody, the things she truly couldn't do for herself.

Using a stove was problematic for Cody. Her difficulty with balance made it dangerous for her to pick up a pan full of hot water or a pot of soup. Her inability to reach anything higher than thirty inches above her head made it hard to access most things in the upper kitchen cabinets, bathroom, closet shelves, a few electrical outlets, and the microwave oven. (Ernie later removed the screws that held it under the upper kitchen cabinet and put it on the counter.) The washers in the building's laundry room were top loading—an odd choice, I thought, for a residence designed to house people in wheelchairs. Cody could not see or reach far enough into the washers to remove clean clothes. She couldn't balance on a shower chair, so she sat on the shower floor to bathe. However, the handle that turned the water on and off was unreachable from the floor. The bedroom was not large enough for Cody to wheel around the entire bed, so changing sheets was a challenge. She couldn't carry a full bag of groceries home from the store and wheel herself at the same time. Nor could she lift a bag of trash into the tall dumpster at the apartment building. There was a long list of everyday things that Cody had trouble with or could not do. Attendant help was a genuine need.

After the nurse left I had a long talk with Cody about the realities of government funding. "If you tell the county folks that you don't need help, they won't provide help. You can see there are quite a few things that you need help with, right?"

Sober now, Cody answered, "Okay, I get it."

Agencies that provided PCAs had to be licensed and approved by the county. A friend in the building recommended the company Cody chose. An agency representative came to the apartment to find out what specific help she needed. Cody explained, "I only want female attendants. I'm not comfortable with strange men helping me with personal things."

The lady from the agency said she couldn't guarantee that. If Cody's PCA was sick or had an emergency, the backup might be a male. "But if that happens, don't worry; these men are used to doing very personal things for female clients. You don't need to feel embarrassed."

Cody remained adamant that she preferred women PCAs. Her first was a woman who also worked with another resident in the building. The PCA came each morning and returned at dinnertime. Different PCAs came on weekends, and sometimes the attendant was someone Cody hadn't met before. Those with years of experience were her favorites. She said, "I like the grandmother-types the best."

Cody's biggest challenge was supervising and directing the work of her PCAs. She had to learn how to best ask for help, describe what she needed, and talk about subjects that involved intimate contact.

Being a PCA was not a high-paying occupation. There was a range of individuals involved in the field. Some people sent to help Cody were compassionate, hardworking folks. Occasionally, an attendant was a nursing student or in training for another medical profession. A part-time job as a PCA was a natural fit with school schedules and caretaking personalities. Those young women, and in one case a young man, were attentive, and Cody became easily attached to them. The relationships often crossed over into friendships. Such was the case with a beautiful young woman named Heather.

When Tad invited Cody to Philadelphia, Heather flew with her. They stayed in a hotel, went to restaurants and plays with Tad and visited his family. Cody cried when Heather left the agency to further her career. There were promises to get together and stay friends, but that didn't happen. Cody learned over time that this type of loss was to be expected.

Some PCAs were unreliable, showed up as much as three hours late, or not at all. Some made long phone calls, helped themselves to food and drinks in her refrigerator, or fell asleep on her couch. Cody had PCAs who stole her money, clothing, CDs, and videos. More than once she called me at work from the phone in her bedroom, speaking in a low voice, to tell me that a PCA was sitting at the kitchen table reading the paper, or her PCA wouldn't do anything Cody asked of her. She was not sure what to do when things like that happened. I helped her think of possible things to say. Mostly I wanted her to protect herself.

Cody was especially anxious when a new PCA came who'd not been interviewed by the agency except by telephone. One such PCA was so uncooperative and unfriendly that Cody left her in the apartment and went to a friend's place to call the agency and me. She didn't return alone to her apartment until the woman left. The agency sent a substitute if one was available, but more often, in this and in many other circumstances, I left work to help Cody myself.

She was afraid to confront dishonest attendants or those with drug and/or alcohol problems or severe mental illness. Cody was threatened on a couple of occasions and once had to call the police when a fired PCA tried to push in her door. There was a ring of PCAs in her building, a mother, her daughters and cousins, who worked interchangeably. It was discovered that they double- and triple-billed more than one agency for the same hours.

After several uncomfortable interchanges with unstable or unscrupulous PCAs, Cody was acutely aware of her vulnerability. I began to drop by to meet her new attendants. Ernie stopped by unannounced from time to time during PCA shifts. Cody bought a lockbox for her cash, checkbook, credit card, and other valuables. She kept it in a kitchen cabinet and put the key on a ring attached to her wheelchair seatbelt. On a day Cody was sick in bed, one PCA pulled Cody's wheelchair into the living room "to get it out of the way" she said. Cody later discovered that money was missing from her lockbox. She didn't like to be suspicious of others, but she learned the hard way that she had to pay close attention when people came to her apartment. With all the things that could be scary, frustrating, or inconvenient when dealing with these individuals, Cody and her friends and neighbors with disabilities placed high value on the help of a kind, honest PCA who allowed them to feel safe at home. The search was always on for such a person who did not move on after a few days, weeks, or months.

In the spring, Ernie and I took Cody on a road trip to visit her cousins in Missouri. Julie took Cody for a ride in her Jeep with the top down. The girls wore matching shirts and their hair blew in all directions as they sped away—two single girls with no particular destination, riding around town on a beautiful warm evening. They played loud music and Cody surprised Julie by knowing the same songs. They screamed the words to music by Michael W. Smith, DC Talk, boy bands, pop, and country music. At stoplights, they quieted down and smiled at guys in cars next to them. The cousins felt wild and free and laughed at each other's jokes. Julie taught Cody the "Jeep wave." Feeling like part of a secret society, Cody held two fingers low on the outside of the passenger door when another Jeep was in sight.

Julie's brother Zach, now seventeen, was tall, athletic, and handsome. He sang and made up his own rap music for special occasions, or any-time really, to amuse the family. Cody asked him to sing again and again. From that visit forward, Cody asked Zach to sing to her by telephone. She said, "Zach's so cute. If he weren't my cousin, I'd marry him."

Chapter 22

Dating

CODY REQUESTED a new computer for her twenty-second birthday. She wanted to surf the Internet and download games. Ernie, now in a computer-related job, found a new PC for her at an auction. She gave her old computer to an attendant. Cody now spent hours surfing the Net, playing games, and honing her typing skills in hopes of finding another office job. Now when we chatted on the phone, I heard her keyboard clicking as she played early generation games like *Ms. Pac-Man, Slingo,* or *Where in the World Is Carmen Santiago?*

The Internet made it possible for all kinds of people to meet each other without physical appearance affecting their first impressions—an important issue to those who know how it feels to be judged and misjudged due to physical differences. This served as a great equalizer for people with disabilities. The Internet widened Cody's world, and her circle of friends multiplied. Talking to others with disabilities, she asked and answered questions on topics that might have embarrassed her to discuss in person. Ernie and I first learned about chatrooms from Cody.

At Thanksgiving, Ernie and I took Cody to Pittsburgh to see Mom. In the eleven months Cody had been living in her own place, she'd gained weight. Even with the doors off the hinges, her new wheelchair didn't fit through Mom's doorways. The first morning, Cody scooted from the bedroom toward her wheelchair in the hall. Ernie had often lifted Cody into her chair if needed; but this time, he couldn't. I knelt on one side of Cody and together we struggled to lift her. The three of us barked instructions to each other as we pulled and floundered in different directions. Cody shouted, "Everybody *stop!*"

While we were frustrated and annoyed with each other, Mom came into the hall and said, "Move over; I'll pick her up." Not that Mom was feeble by any means even at age eighty-six, but the idea that she could lift 140 pounds, which we together couldn't, made us all laugh. Undaunted, Mom reached under Cody's arms with complete confidence. Despite Cody's willingness to be lifted, she remained firmly seated on the floor. "Oh my!" Mom frowned.

"It's okay," I said, "we'll go back to basics." We used the old wheelbarrow technique, lifting Cody's ankles as she crawled forward on her elbows. She pulled herself onto the living room couch and into her wheelchair. I untangled her legs as she turned around in the seat, and this method worked for the remainder of our stay.

I worried about Cody's weight increase as it became harder for her to move around and do things for herself. Her breathing was strained more easily when she exerted herself, and some transfers were more difficult. I was careful to broach the subject only in the context of health and mobility, but she responded with annoyance, "Yeah, yeah, yeah. I know."

Sometime that winter Cody was injured during a transfer from her wheelchair to her bed. The second to smallest toe on her right foot snagged on something and was almost torn off. Cody discovered the injury a day or so later when she saw blood on her sock. Her PCAs bandaged the toe daily for weeks, but by Valentine's Day her doctor was concerned that the slow healing could be due to diabetes. A test ruled out diabetes, but Cody's scare lingered.

Cody called later that night. "Hey, Mom, that doctor almost ruined Valentine's Day . . . but my day *improved*." A man had asked her out on a date—a "real" date she said, with a forty-year-old who lived in her building. She sounded like an excited teenager. But after her dinner date, Cody decided they'd probably just be friends.

By late April an infection had developed in Cody's toe. When the doctor said it had to be amputated, Cody sobbed. Her eyes flashed. "I'll look like a freak without a toe!"

I tried to convince her that losing a toe was not such a big deal, but I truly shared Cody's sadness and anger. Few parts of my daughter's body were untouched by injury or surgery of some kind: her head, neck, back, legs, abdomen, feet, and now her toe. Loss of a toe was not life-threatening, but it was yet another loss. I told Cody how sorry I was and added, "At least you won't need anesthesia since you can't feel your foot."

She brightened a little, then whimpered, "I'll never be able to wear sandals again."

Cody asked Ernie to be with her for the day surgery. He held her hand and distracted her from the procedure. I was grateful. I didn't want to watch or, more to the point, try not to watch.

Cody's favorite PCA resigned that same week and a guy she had a crush on moved out of the building. I felt so sad for her losses and worried that she was depressed. Two days after the toe amputation, I stopped by with a cheer-up gift. Cody was sitting at her kitchen table, her bandaged foot resting on the raised pedal of her wheelchair.

I had again underestimated Cody's resilience. She was in high spirits. Her eyes sparkled as she grinned. "Look at this!"

Cody had sculpted a small toe with flour and water, and painted it to look real. It stuck out of a piece of gauze stained with red food coloring tucked into a clear plastic culture tube. The hospital sticker with Cody's name was taped to the tube. As I looked closely at the fake toe, Cody said, "I'm going to send it to Dad in Hawaii with a note that says: Since you can't be here with me, I'm sending a little part of me to be with you." We both burst out laughing.

Still giggling, she said, "My new attendant thinks it's gross."

"Well, yeah," I agreed, "it's amazing. It looks real."

Cody kept laughing as she told me about her friends' reactions. "Half of them think it's a totally funny thing to send Dennis. The rest think I'm a sick-o."

I offered, "Hey, I have some stuff we could use to make a toenail. I'll bring it tomorrow after work. Then we'll mail it to Dennis."

Cody said, "Cool." We kept laughing and imagining Dennis's reaction.

The following day, the fake toe was missing. We searched every possible place in Cody's apartment, but the toe was gone. She suspected that her new PCA threw it in the dumpster. Just as we gave up the search, Tad called to confirm his visit in May. Cody told him about her aborted plan to send a fake toe to Dennis on sabbatical in Hawaii.

Tad said, "Cody! That is so gross. Don't you *ever* do anything like that to me! *Ewww!*"

Cody laughed again and said, "You just don't understand my relationship with Dennis. He'd think it was funny."

Tad insisted, "No way, Cody. That is *too* gross!"

After she hung up, Cody giggled and said, "And I thought he was the *fun* father."

Dennis later told Cody that he probably would have been grossed out at first, but then he would have thought it was really funny.

Cody said, "I knew it."

Cody had a bad cold in September. I called at bedtime to see how she was feeling. She said in a stuffy voice, "I don't feel too good."

"Do you have a fever?"

"No. I'm just clogged up. I took some vitamin C and had a cup of tea."

"Okay then, sweet dreams, babe. Say your prayers."

At 2:00 a.m. the phone rang, and I jumped to grab it. Cody said in alarm, "Mom, I can't breathe! Come right away!" and hung up.

I dialed her number quickly and she answered, crying.

"Cody, tell me what's wrong!" I couldn't understand her answer through her sobs and gasps. I spoke strongly, "Cody! Talk to me! If you can't breath, we need to call 9-1-1."

"No!" Her voice shuddered as she tried to stop crying. "I'm okay. I just need help."

"Are you sure you're okay?"

She cried, "Yeah, I'm okay. I'm just having trouble. I can't find my inhaler, and my bed's wet. I want you to come."

As my panic dissolved, I spoke in anger. "Listen, Cody, I will come. But don't you *ever* call and say something like you can't breathe and hang up! Besides, you don't need to freak out to get me to help you. Just be truthful about what's wrong, okay?"

She whimpered, "You're coming now?"

"Yes. I'm getting dressed. I'll be there in fifteen minutes."

"Thanks, Mom."

By the time I arrived at Cody's apartment, she was in her wheelchair. Her eyelashes were still wet with tears, but she felt fine. I found her inhaler in a drawer beside her bed amidst vitamin bottles, snack-food wrappers, makeup, and craft supplies. She took a puff. We had a serious talk while I changed her sheets. I used a stern voice to bring home my point. "Cody. I really mean this. I *never* want you to call at two in the morning, or any time, to tell me you can't breathe! I mean it, Cody. You need to dial 9-1-1 *immediately* if you can't breathe. I can't get here as fast as an ambulance. And *I* can't help you breathe if you're really in trouble. I want you to get *real* help when you need it. I need to know that you understand what I'm saying."

"I do. I will. I'll call 9-1-1 first, if I really can't breathe."

"Promise me."

Cody looked up at me sincerely and said, "I promise." She rolled from her wheelchair back into bed and I kissed her.

She said, "I'm sorry you had to come in the middle of the night."

"That's okay, sweetie. I'm glad you're feeling better. Keep taking vitamin C for your cold. And drink lots of water tomorrow."

"Okay."

Two weeks later, the phone rang again at 2:00 a.m. and my heart skipped a beat.

Cody spoke fast, "Hi Mom! I'm fine! I just couldn't wait until morning to tell you. I just made out with a guy! I just had my first truly romantic kissing."

"That's great, babe." I tried to wake up enough to talk more. "Is he still there with you?"

Her enthusiasm barely contained, she said, "No, he just left."

"Are you okay?"

"Oh, yeah! We made out for a couple of hours! It was great!"

"That's terrific, sweetie. I'm really glad you had a good time. Is it okay if you tell me the details when I'm more awake?"

"All right!" Cody added a little squeal and said, "I'll call you in the morning."

I hung up the phone. Ernie was almost awake, looking at me. "Is she okay?"

"Yeah. She made out with a guy; she's excited." Ernie fell back to sleep almost instantly. But I lay awake thinking how happy Cody sounded and how grateful I felt that she still wanted to tell me her good news. I almost called her right back to hear the details.

The instant I arrived at work in the morning, the phone rang. Cody told me more about the guy. He was forty-one; he had cerebral palsy. Most of the kissing took place while both of them sat in their wheelchairs. Cody added, "He's not really handsome, but he's really sweet. He's coming over again tonight. I can't wait."

I asked how she met him. Cody gushed on like she had in high school when describing boys she liked. "He was a friend of the guy in the building who I used to have a crush on. I hung out a lot with them. Here I was, gaga over my friend, and all the time this guy was gaga over me! I couldn't believe it!"

He had come over to watch a movie with Cody and turned off the lights so the atmosphere felt like a movie theater. He moved closer and closer until his arm was around her. Cody said, "When he started to kiss me, I stopped him for a second. I asked if he was going to do the tongue thing. He said 'No' and I said 'That's good, because I have to warn you, I have a powerful gag reflex.'"

I laughed and teased Cody about gagging not being too sexy.

Her date wanted to sleep with her, but Cody told him, "Not yet." She set some ground rules. He said that he'd only do things she was comfortable with; he wouldn't rush her in any way. "So we kissed and kissed for hours. My jaw is tired."

"Was your mouth closed tight the whole time while you kissed?"

"Yeah."

I told Cody how proud I was that she set boundaries, and that she did only what she wanted to do with her new boyfriend. "And, I have a tip for you when you kiss him tonight. Relax your lips and let them feel soft.

Part your lips just a little. You can move your lips around some while you're kissing."

Cody called first thing the next morning. "Mom! That kissing tip was the best! It made a big difference. He said I'm the best kisser he's ever had."

Two weeks later her new boyfriend told her he never wanted to leave her. Cody wrote him a letter explaining more details about her disability so that he knew what to expect from her if they became more intimate.

She said, "I thought if I tried to talk to him about it, I'd get flustered and forget what I was saying."

Cody had often asked if I'd ever marry Ernie, and I finally gave her the news she was waiting for. She screamed, "Yay! Now I'll have three dads— like *Three Men and a Little Lady!*"

Ernie and I flew to Las Vegas to be married in December. But while we were gone, Cody suffered a broken heart. Her forty-one-year-old turned out to be "immature." After their two months as a couple, he told her, "I screwed up. I'm sorry. I can't handle commitment." But even as he said this, he told Cody that she was beautiful and repeated that she was the best kisser he'd ever had, and the best sex (despite the fact that their physical interactions had not included intercourse). As Cody described her heartbreak, I thought again how the hardest part about being a parent is when the kid hurts, no matter what the reason or how old the kid is.

Despite occasional rejections, Cody remained a hopeful romantic. She told me about every cute guy she liked and provided details about whatever intimacies she experienced. I was her happy girlfriend, enjoying her enthusiasm and commiserating with her disappointments.

Whenever she told Dennis about her boyfriends, he didn't want details. "I don't want to think of some man pawing my daughter."

This gave Cody license to tease him. She took delight in seeing Dennis squirm when she mentioned anything about kissing or sex.

Cody met several young men in chatrooms on the Internet and had fun flirting with them online. Ernie warned Cody about online predators and cautioned her not to reveal her last name, address, or phone number to new online friends.

Irish musicians played violin, mandolin, guitar, and bodhran at our house party in June to celebrate our marriage. My mother greeted guests at the door, and Cody chatted with everyone. Her cousin Joanna sat at the piano with Ernie's nephews. My brother danced with Ernie's sister.

Cody said to Lorraine, "Now you're my new grandmother," and Lorraine smiled, saying, "Yes." Before a Metro Mobility bus took Cody home, she called me into the bedroom. She gave me a charm in the shape of a house and said, "I'm so happy you married Ernie."

She had referred to Ernie as "Mom's boyfriend" for more than two years. Now she called him her stepdad, but introduced us to friends and PCAs as her parents without the "step" part. She made a giant card for him on Father's Day that said she was happy to have him as a dad.

When Cody turned twenty-four in August, a dozen red roses in a cobalt-blue glass vase were delivered to my office at work with the note: "To the greatest mom in the world. Happy 24th Anniversary of the birth of your baby girl! I love you, Cody."

In October, after three years with the same agency, Cody was fed up with unreliable PCAs who left the company, got married, had babies, followed boyfriends out of town, went into chemical dependency treatment, or gave any number of other reasons for leaving after a few days or weeks. Some new health problems made reliable help from PCAs more essential. I joined Cody when the nurse from the new agency came to interview her. Cody described a typical day and included her health issues.

As she'd done since childhood, Cody rolled out of bed in the morning and sat on the floor to cath herself. She lifted sideways on her right hip to push down to empty her bowels. Her stool was usually firm and came out in tidy manageable pieces. After emptying her bowels as best she could, she used moist wipes, then wrapped the incontinent brief for disposal. She scooted into the bathroom where she sat on the floor to take her morning shower.

Antibiotics were prescribed every few weeks due to more frequent urinary tract infections. Cody recognized a UTI by a sudden strong smell from her urine or an otherwise unexplained fever. Because Cody often coughed hard and gasped with colds, asthma had been added to her medical summary. More antibiotics were prescribed a few times a year for this. Refusing allergy medication that made her drowsy or dizzy, she instead found an over-the-counter alternative to use along with her inhaler.

The agency nurse noticed that Cody's ankles and feet were swollen. This was something new. Her primary care doctor thought it was due to poor circulation. He had advised Cody to elevate her legs for part of each day. She had discovered pressure sores on the heels of both feet that now required daily wound care. After the nurse left I read the care plan summary:

> PCA to assist with Activities of Daily Living: Make meals, refrigerate for Cody to warm up. She needs to eat healthy foods high in protein to promote healing of ulcers. PCA to help with dressing if Cody is ill. Cody does her own bathing, shampooing, showering, and drying. Cody refuses help with peri care. Some movement difficulty due to weight and edema. Using Keflex, Proventl puffs, Claritin as needed. Allergy to cold. Gets on floor in shower. Hours: 10–1 , 4–6.

PCAs from the new agency were more reliable; Cody was rarely stranded. She called me less often as she became more involved with online friends and the occasional new love interest. I heard from her only once a day and our conversations were shorter. I took this as a healthy indication that she had a life, and she was busy living it.

Ernie and I stopped by her place a couple of times a week. Cody played her favorite new songs for us and introduced us to new PCAs or someone she was dating. We met Jake, who had cerebral palsy. He had an accessible wheelchair van, which meant they could go places together. The relationship involved a lot of laughing, from what I could tell. Jake had his attendant take pictures of him reclining naked in various poses as a gift for Cody. One afternoon, Cody giggled and showed me the pictures. Ernie was busy checking expiration dates and throwing away outdated food from Cody's refrigerator. I winked to Cody as I handed the pictures to Ernie.

Ernie, distracted by his project when he took the stack of pictures, glanced at the photos in his hands, recoiled with a start, and said, "Whoa. I didn't need to see this."

Cody dissolved into laughter. Ernie said, "Jake probably didn't intend for you to show these to anyone."

With a wide smile Cody said, "Why not? He looks pretty good, don't you think?" She collapsed laughing again.

Cody exchanged emails for some time with Frank from Wisconsin. He drove three hours to meet her. She made sure she had a friend present the first time he came. Frank was a sweet guy, attentive, and offered to help with some of her personal cares. But after a few trips, Cody discouraged him from further visits. He called on and off for the next year asking to come back, but Cody was firm in her view that she and Frank had no future.

Cody had a romantic date with a man she'd known for a few years. Matt was in an electric-powered wheelchair. Instead of breathing through his nose and mouth, he had a tracheostomy tube that went into his windpipe through an opening in his throat. He and Cody were solid friends with an attraction that they finally acted upon one night. They kissed with enthusiasm and, without realizing it, Cody yanked out his breathing tube. Matt wasn't disturbed by this accident; he simply called his attendant in from the next room to replace the tube. He was fine, but Cody was horrified. She told Matt she was sorry but they couldn't continue an intimate relationship. He tried to convince her otherwise, but she was definite about it.

She told me, "I could have *killed* him!"

I said, "It sounds like it was no big deal for him. You don't want a minor accident to keep you from someone you really care about, right?"

"No way, Mom! I'm too scared I'd hurt him."

Chapter 23

Blooming

SEVEN YEARS WITHOUT a medical emergency ended when Cody developed pressure behind her eyes and a severe and worsening headache in March 1997. She was directed to United Hospital, across from her neurosurgeon's St. Paul office. Symptoms of a shunt problem subsided within hours, but a full health history and physical with lab tests revealed three "potentially life-threatening" medical conditions.

Cody had a virulent urinary tract infection that had shown no noticeable symptoms. The "exotic" bacteria strain was resistant to the antibiotic she'd taken for years. Cody admitted that for some months she'd found her incontinent briefs wet no matter how often she cathed herself. She was now entirely unable to stay dry. As a result, her skin had broken down. She had not felt the "extensive skin ulcerations on her buttocks and lower sacrum." The skin was gone from the entire surface of both of her butt cheeks. The sight was disturbing.

At the hospital that evening, Cody, Dennis, Ernie, and I listened to the attending physician explain Cody's conditions and proposed treatments. The rampant bladder infection required immediate IV antibiotics. Due to a severe iron deficiency anemia, she had to be given a unit of packed red blood cells. The physician said any one of the situations with her skin lesions, blood, or UTI could have been life threatening. Each had been caught just in time. I saw fear in Cody's eyes as he spoke.

She was transferred to a Rehab floor once she was medically stable. She had to lie in sideways positions to avoid pressure on her buttocks. Layers of medicated mesh were put on her wounds. A Foley catheter inserted into her urethra kept the area dry. The skin lesions needed careful monitoring to prevent infection; Cody was to be in the hospital for several weeks. A new wheelchair was prescribed with customized seating and back support, and a dietician was consulted. A psychiatric evaluation was ordered after all of the above, not surprisingly, caused Cody a good deal of anxiety.

A new practice began in the hospital: digital stool removal. A nurse wore a vinyl glove and reached one or two fingers into Cody's rectum to assist with bowel movements. This method made sure her bowels were emptied completely. Cody had to get used to the idea of allowing a PCA to do this each morning.

Cody's latex allergy was confirmed—hence the vinyl, rather than latex, gloves. Hospitals had begun to take latex allergies seriously as healthcare workers and patients with long-term exposure developed sensitivities and adverse health effects. There were reports of anaphylactic reactions and deaths. People with spina bifida were prime candidates for latex allergies due to recurring contact during hospitalizations and daily use of equipment such as latex catheters.

Though Cody had not used latex catheters for some time, her symptoms of latex sensitivity had been going on for years. She had noticed that her hands itched and her throat felt tight when she touched balloons or pencil erasers. Natural rubber proteins were also in many foods. I recalled her extreme reaction to eating a peach a few years before. Her entire face swelled. Cody was cautioned to avoid more of her favorites like bananas and avocados. Her nurses used latex-free Foley catheters and blood pressure cuffs. A cart with latex-free medical supplies and equipment was parked in the corner of her hospital room. Wound dressings were checked first for latex. If nurses were unsure about a product, Ernie called the manufacturer.

As I added latex to the allergy portion of Cody's medical summary, I wondered if latex caused Cody's occasional breathing distress. I cringed to think of all the latex she was exposed to throughout her childhood. I knew that I, like most mothers, did the best I could with what I knew as I raised my daughter. But I still felt that horrible cringe whenever I learned new information about something during her childhood that resulted in long-term or permanent harm.

Ernie and I went to Cody's apartment to pick up her mail and search for items containing latex. We found Band-Aids, rubber bands, art erasers, kitchen utensils with rubber parts, rubber gloves for cleaning, Koosh balls, Ace bandages, art glue, chewing gum, adhesive tapes, and elastic waistbands in her clothing. Latex was everywhere, even in the tires of her wheelchair.

Cody was reluctant to speak with a psychiatrist. She told me, "I'm afraid he'll try to force me to take medication. I don't want to feel drugged. It reminds me of surgery and anesthesia. I'd rather be anxious."

The psychiatrist arrived unannounced one morning in her room. After he left, Cody requested a copy of his report. The doctor wrote that Cody was "pleasant and cooperative, of average intelligence with a good fund of knowledge, a mild voice tremor, good eye contact, and able to smile and joke." He said her "insight into her illness is good" and quoted Cody's initial comments: "I know a lot about my anxiety. It's panic disorder, and fear of places. I have a therapist, and I have to tell you that medicines don't interest me."

I recognized Cody's strong language—*I have to tell you*—regarding medication. That's probably when he heard the "mild voice tremor." I could tell she stuck up for herself in the interview. The "History of Present Illness" portion recounted Cody's struggle with anxiety:

> The patient is a delightful Caucasian female who presents in a very frank way. She describes having anxiety since age seven. This in the context of memories of being medically disabled and having significant fears about whether she would live or not. She states she has frequent memories of her initial anxiety, which was related to hospitalization, and frequently feels worse in regard to anxiety, either when being left alone or when in the hospital. She feels this worry has improved with time, but she is quite aware of panic. "I used to have to make myself go out." Currently she rarely has significant panic, perhaps every month or so. Although she has anxiety about going out in public, she continues to leave as often as needed. She denies symptoms consistent with other anxiety disorders or depression.

Diagnostic impression:

(1) Panic Disorder with agoraphobia, in partial remission

(2) R/O [rule out] resolving PTSD from childhood medical trauma.

Under "Recommendations" he wrote that Cody might benefit from pharmacological intervention for her panic, but that she was "unwilling to consider it at this time."

Cody asked me, "What's PTSD?"

"Posttraumatic stress disorder. It's what happens to some people after a very upsetting experience. He thinks your anxiety may be related to a scary experience when you were little that still bothers you. Maybe something that happened in the hospital."

"Like when they put that mask over my face in the operating room?"

"Right."

After six days in the hospital, Cody's shunt malfunction symptoms returned. A CAT scan confirmed intracranial pressure. The neurosurgeon was able to press on the soft spot over her shunt to pump it, so he decided against surgery for the time being.

Cody asked him, "Are you sure I'm okay? Is there any chance I might arrest tonight like I did when I was fifteen?"

The doctor said, "I can't tell you for sure that there is no chance, but I'm quite comfortable that there is a relatively small chance of that."

After he left, Cody said, "Well, I'm glad *he's* comfortable. I can't say *I* am."

Cody's intuition was on alert, and her concerns were affirmed when the morning nurse had difficulty waking her. Her headache had returned. Her eyes were sunsetting, and she was slightly nauseous. She was taken to the operating room for a shunt revision.

After the operation I wiped excess surgical soap out of Cody's hair with a wet washcloth. Dennis spent the night with her. Cody called late to say goodnight.

I asked, "How are you, sweetie?"

"Dad fainted."

"Did he watch a nurse take your blood?"

"Yeah."

"Is he okay, now?"

"Yeah, he's lying on a cot next to me. He moans once in a while. The nurse brought him some juice."

Cody was transferred back to the Rehab floor two days after her shunt surgery. She said she felt like her "old self" again. Nurses helped her change position frequently from face down to sideways without disturbing the wounds. Cody did not complain about her restricted movement. She listened to music on her headset and showed Ernie how to macramé bracelets with colored twine. Ernie and I stayed each night until bedtime and one of us returned in the morning. My brother Charlie called her almost daily; her cousin Zachary sang songs over the phone. Cody requested a visit from the hospital's spiritual services department. When asked if she preferred a priest, minister, or rabbi, she chose all three.

The wound care specialist assessed the healing of Cody's butt each morning. After several days, the clinician was excited.

"This is very good. We have buds!"

Cody asked, "Buds?" I moved closer as the clinician pointed to several rounded half-inch areas on the raw surface that looked like thin membranes. I saw what she meant, but it was a long way from looking like skin.

The specialist continued, "As more of these buds appear, the areas widen. Layers of skin will grow up from underneath. This is good news."

Cody said, "Well, I'm glad my butt's blooming."

After almost a month on the hospital Rehab floor, Cody was allowed to go home. She was given self-care instructions before discharge. Her PCAs were to continue wound care. She was counseled on reproductive health and skin care in her perineal area during sexual activity. She was advised to use lubrication during sex to prevent skin breakdown, and use a mirror following intercourse to check skin for injury. Though Cody, at twenty-four, had not engaged in sexual intercourse, I was glad somebody was *finally* providing practical information about sex for a woman with a disability.

Cody requested copies of her medical summaries after she left the hospital. She was concerned that the rehab physician included several inaccuracies and misspelled Cody's last name. The error that most bothered her was that the doctor wrote that Cody had a VP (rather than VA) shunt. VP (ventriculoperitoneal) shunts directed cerebrospinal fluid from the brain ventricle through tubing that extends to the abdomen. VA (ventriculoatrial) shunts were directed into the vascular system (a vein) to the heart. Tests and surgical procedures differed for each. For a shunt scan, radiology technicians x-rayed more of her body if they thought she had a VP shunt (to include the lower abdomen). Cody tried to avoid unnecessary x-rays. She wrote a letter requesting that errors be corrected in her hospital record. She was told she could add a letter with corrections but hospital rules forbade removal of information from the chart "even if it's wrong."

I had read Cody's medical chart periodically and was amazed at how frequently I found wrong information. I doubted that busy doctors actually read supplemental letters, or even noticed them in a chart as thick as Cody's.

The hospital discharge summary suggested a urology consult to consider surgical options to address Cody's incontinence now that she had a "flaccid urethral sphincter." Keeping her skin dry was essential. But Cody didn't want to think about surgery.

Ernie constructed a rolling platform so Cody wouldn't drag her butt across the floor between her bedroom and bathroom. She now transferred from her bed to the floor in the mornings and slid easily onto the platform. Her PCA pulled her with the attached strap like a sled on wheels to and from the bathroom.

Cody's new skin was so delicate that even removing paper tape could tear it. Several times, a PCA pulled tape off quickly and the healing had to begin again. I now showed every PCA how to dress the wounds. For several months I went to Cody's apartment once or twice a day to change dressings. If I was at work, Ernie picked up wound care supplies, helped her change clothes, or fixed her bandages if they came apart. Cody soon realized how hard it was to keep her wounds dry and prevent further skin breakdown. She finally agreed to hear about surgical solutions for dealing with incontinence.

The urologist didn't smile or make any obvious attempt to help Cody feel comfortable as he described a procedure called Augmentation Cystoplasty with Mitrofanoff. He directed his conversation to Ernie and me and spoke in technical terms as though lecturing medical students. In fact, he ignored Cody as though she wasn't even in the room. In a sense, she wasn't. I saw a look of tuned-out panic on her face. Ernie and I listened to the mechanical discourse and asked questions to understand risks and details. Cody remained silent and stared at the door.

Basically, the surgery involved an incision from the naval to the pubic area. A piece of bowel would be patched to the bladder to enlarge its capacity. The bladder would be rerouted to a new opening at the naval instead of the urethra. A straw-like tube several inches long (called a Mitrofanoff) would be refashioned from her appendix. Cody could insert a catheter into the new opening at her bellybutton to empty her bladder. The Mitrofanoff was designed to collapse internally to a squashed Z, called a flap valve, so leakage didn't occur between catheterizations. Paul Mitrofanoff was the inventor of the procedure, first used in 1980.

The idea of a permanent change in the configuration of internal organs sounded bizarre and troubling. I fully understood why Cody tuned out. She didn't speak until we were in the hall waiting for the elevator. She looked up at Ernie, then at me.

In a stern and measured voice she said, "I have one thing to say— *second opinion!*"

I laughed. "I agree. It sounds pretty weird. But it would be neat to be able to cath yourself without getting out of your chair. We may have to get over how weird it sounds and think of the advantages. This surgery may be our only solution."

When Cody was a child, I explained to her why an operation was for her own good, why she didn't have a choice. But now she made the decisions. I knew that if she didn't go through with it, we'd each have to live with the consequences. This surgery could make Cody's life easier in so many ways—no more multiple transfers from wheelchair to bed to floor in order to cath herself, and no more inability to be out for more than two hours. She'd be able to cath herself almost anywhere. The procedure offered freedom. But it sounded scary.

Cody conducted her own research. She contacted Internet friends and talked to others with spina bifida who either considered or had bladder augmentation. Her fingers flew on the keyboard as she gathered opinions from around the country.

She discussed her fears about the surgery with her new psychotherapist, Mab. Though I never met Mab, I could tell she was the right therapist for Cody. It spoke volumes to me that she remembered things Mab said. Cody had more self-confidence. I rarely heard the timid voice tremor mentioned by the hospital psychiatrist.

I arranged for the second opinion Cody requested. Joe Lee was a soft-spoken urologist who'd been at Gillette Hospital since his residency. Cody liked him. Dr. Lee presented the same information as the first urologist, but he spoke directly to Cody. He emphasized how the surgery could improve the quality of her life. The whole idea didn't seem nearly as creepy to me or, more importantly, to Cody.

She asked, "How many times have you done this operation?"

Dr. Lee said he'd done it several times and offered to have Cody speak with his other patients. He described postoperative complications that one or two people had, and said what he'd do to prevent those for Cody.

"What about my weight? Is the operation dangerous since I'm overweight?"

"You're a little round," Dr. Lee answered in gentle voice, "but that won't matter. You'll be fine. That's not a problem."

Cody asked, "Can I get my tubes tied at the same time?"

Dr. Lee nodded. "That's possible. You can talk to a gynecologist about that."

Cody had decided she didn't want to have children, but most birth control methods were not options. Her latex allergy ruled out rubber diaphragms and most condoms. She didn't want to take pills with hormones that might alter her moods. The ability to have a tubal ligation while she was already in surgery provided her with more incentive to have the bladder operation. After doing her own research and talking again to Dr. Lee, Cody was still unsure.

She turned to Ernie and asked, "What do you think?"

Ernie hadn't expressed an opinion, but he'd been involved in all meetings and discussions with the doctors. He told Cody, "If it was me, I'd have the surgery. You'll be able go out for longer periods of time."

After his brief comment Cody scheduled surgery for the fall.

As summer months passed, Cody kept me abreast of her Internet romance with a guy thirteen years older. John's name came up daily while I dressed her wounds. "He wants me to come to California to meet his family. After the bladder operation, I could travel easier. He asked me to marry him, but I don't have a ring, yet."

At first I assumed John was another lucky recipient of Cody's easy affection. By fall, as she prepared to undergo the lengthy bladder augmentation surgery, I saw how special their cyberspace relationship had become. John had encouraged her to go ahead with the surgery. I suspected his support helped her maintain her bravery once the decision was made. He sent Cody a picture of himself in a wheelchair next to a cedar tree. In a letter he wrote, "I'm glad you are so accepting of me. A lot of women can't deal with my combination of disabilities. I don't want to lose you or drift apart. I love you very much, you are the best."

I asked Cody, "John looks in pretty good shape. Why does he use a wheelchair?"

She said, "He has CP and he's legally blind. He can walk with crutches, but it's hard for him to go too far without his wheelchair."

Although he lived with his parents, John sounded fairly independent. He loved camping, had a job with the phone company, and had traveled to Europe a few times with friends. Cody had other friends with cerebral palsy, such as Sharon. I had trouble understanding some of them, so I asked Cody, "Is his speech affected by his CP?"

"Nope, he talks fine." Cody went on about how cute and sweet John was.

A month before Cody's bladder surgery, her friend Gertrude called from an inpatient mental health unit. She had been admitted to the hospital with suicidal depression.

Gertrude and Cody had become friends when they sat across from each other in Mr. Debe's tenth grade creative writing class. A few boys in the back of the room picked on Gertrude, and Cody told them to shut up. "Cody tells it like it is," Gertrude told me.

Gertrude was about to be released from the hospital. A social worker had given her a list of transitional housing options, but Gertrude had to make the calls. She told Cody, "I don't know what to do. I need to find somewhere to live. I don't want to go back home. It's not a healthy place for me right now."

Cody said firmly, "You're coming home with me. *I'll* take care of you."

Gertrude moved into Cody's apartment and slept on the sofabed. Cody told her she could stay as long as she needed. Each morning before Gertrude left for her aftercare day-treatment program, Cody packed a lunch for her, set up the medications a psychiatrist prescribed for Gertrude and reminded her when to take them. The girls watched videos together in the evenings or visited Cody's friend Oscar in his apartment on the second floor. If they ate out, Cody paid for the meals. Three weeks later, Gertrude was accepted into a supportive group environment with others in similar circumstances.

Cody told me John wanted to know if he could send her email messages to my work address while she was in the hospital. I asked, "Won't he mind your mother seeing his private emails to you?"

Cody said no, he'd be fine with that.

The evening before the operation Cody was in bed for the night at Gillette Hospital. She was nervous about surgery and wanted to talk to her Uncle Charlie. We couldn't make long-distance calls from the hospital, so Charlie arranged to call later to say a prayer with Cody. Nurses came and went through the evening, taking blood, temperature, and blood pressure; sorting out wound dressing supplies; and locating the correct catheters. Charlie called as planned; they prayed and talked. John called next. Cody chatted and laughed for several minutes, then said, "John, this is my mother," and handed the phone to me.

John had a strong male voice as he conveyed a sincere caring and concern for Cody. I was impressed with him—impressed with the power he had to help Cody stay calm (at least calmer) in the face of her big operation. He promised to call her after surgery.

Dr. Lee allowed Cody to pick music to be played in the operating room. She brought three CDs. She was also permitted to bring someone with her into the O.R. She paused before deciding and looked up at me with a trace of internal conflict on her face.

I said, "It's okay, Cody. Choose who you really want with you."

"Okay. I want Ernie to come with me."

Ernie put on a white Tyvek bodysuit, blue disposable shoe covers, the bouffant cap, and a facemask. I kissed Cody and leaned close for our usual pre-surgery prayer. Tears welled in my eyes watching Cody and Ernie grip each other's hands as the gurney was wheeled into the operating room.

I felt continually grateful that Ernie loved Cody so much. He did so many things for her that I could not have done and also kept my job. He tried to protect her and make her life more fun. He never seemed to mind interrupting whatever he was doing to help her. He left work to pick her up if she was lost, stuck in the rain, or if she needed help with something in her apartment. He researched products for people with disabilities and read about her medications, vitamins, and allergies. He built new equipment when there was nothing available for what she needed. He took her places and picked up her friends to come along. It made Cody happy that he also spent time just with her, and genuinely enjoyed doing so. He dropped by to bring her new computer games, teach her a new software program, or take her shopping. He often slipped her some cash; she smiled and said thanks. Cody felt safe with Ernie, and I felt the same gratefulness as years before when he first fixed her wheelchair.

Ernie came out of the O.R. fifteen minutes later, looking slightly shaken. He described what had happened next. He'd held Cody's hand and spoken with her for a few minutes as O.R. clinicians bustled around them. The anesthesiologist didn't say anything when he injected the sedative into Cody's IV; Ernie was startled for a moment when he saw her eyes suddenly become vacant and her eyelids half close. The doctor apologized to Ernie for the lack of warning.

Eight hours later, Dennis, Ernie, and I were waiting for Cody when she came out of the recovery room. Her face had the puffiness and waxy look we'd seen often after surgeries, but gradually her color returned. Her abdomen had a long line of black stitches. Although Cody had no sensation over most of the area around the incision, she described feeling a little beat up.

The nurse gave her a clear-blue plastic apparatus called an incentive spirometer. Using its mouthpiece, she inhaled as deeply as possible to make a small plastic ball float up, stimulating coughs to help clear her lungs from anesthesia. Cody inhaled as best she could and her results improved over the next two days.

As promised, John sent daily emails professing his love. Impressed with what he knew so far about John, Dennis offered an airline ticket so Cody and John could meet in person. John had heard that Minnesota winters could be pretty cold, so he made plans to come in the spring.

Chapter 24

Meeting John

By December, Cody was able to appreciate the freedom her surgery promised. She could go to movies again, shop for hours, and cath herself almost anywhere. She decided the bladder operation was a wise choice and spread the word on the Internet to her similarly affected friends. Cody's grandmother, aunts, uncles, and cousins from my family came to the Twin Cities for Christmas. On our last morning together Charlie suggested that each of us share some personal news the rest of us might not already know about the other. When it was Cody's turn, she announced she was engaged to a man she had not yet met. Excitement broke out. Cody's face glowed as everyone congratulated her and asked questions about John.

In the spring, Cody let out a happy squeal as she transferred into the backseat of our car to go to the airport to meet John's flight. She had carefully chosen just the right outfit for their first meeting. Her cheeks reflected the hot-pink top she wore with black cotton pants and black hightops with hot-pink laces. Her hair was shoulder length and brushed back. Her red beaded earrings had pink hearts.

Ernie folded her wheelchair into the trunk along with her backup chair for John's use. John was bringing crutches only; he didn't want the airline to damage his chair. I understood his caution. Cody's had been banged up a few times during air travel, leaving broken wheel spokes, scratched paint, loose brakes, scuffs, and dings.

Cody said, "I'm so excited. I can't wait. I hope he still likes me once he actually sees me."

I said, "How could he not like you, babe? You're terrific, and you look great."

"I love John so much. I decided I don't even mind if he's a drooler."

I hadn't thought of that. Cody and I both were grossed out by excess drool, even though folks with that trouble couldn't help it. Cody sometimes wiped her friend Joe's face. For all we knew, John might be a drooler. I said sincerely, "That's true love, sweetie."

At the airport Cody wheeled ahead to the gate. I assumed John would be last off the plane and was surprised to see him amidst a group of passengers already coming out of the Jetway. He took quick strides, using crutches with metal arm cuffs. He planted the crutches firmly and thrust both legs forward together. Though John was "legally blind," he moved toward us without hesitation. He stopped in front of Cody. She grabbed him by the arm and pulled him down for a tight hug before he exchanged hellos with Ernie and me. John wore glasses, and his right eye turned in slightly. He faced me directly when I spoke.

On the way to the car, John moved as fast on crutches as Cody wheeled her chair. Ernie and I walked faster to keep up with them. After Cody transferred into the car, John stood outside, watching Ernie put her chair in the trunk.

Cody whispered to me, "He's gorgeous!" The smile that appeared on her face when she saw John remained wide and happy all the way home. She leaned against him, hugging his arm. Ernie and I asked about his trip, and Cody and John talked some. He was polite and conversed readily about his family and job. He had two brothers. His family home was in Oakland. At Cody's apartment building, John thanked Ernie for the ride.

Cody's plan was to call later to tell me whether John was as wonderful in person as he was from a distance. I hoped along with her that it was the real thing, but we had discussed the possibility that their feelings might change once they actually spent time together. Mostly, I didn't want Cody to be hurt or disappointed.

A half hour later, she called, speaking in a hushed voice. "He still loves me! He's in the bathroom. He still wants to marry me . . . he says I'm pretty . . . he loves my hair. Gotta go. Bye."

For the next week Cody packed in as much activity as possible. She and John rode Metro Mobility buses to the Mall of America and around town. She arranged for each of her closest girlfriends to meet him. They hung out at Oscar's apartment part of every day. Dennis stopped by to meet John and said he approved—John was "a nice guy."

An easygoing affection took hold of the happy couple. Cody teased John the way she teased her cousin Zachary. John laughed along and teased her back.

After several busy days, Cody began to look tired. I suggested she spend a day at home. But she didn't want to deprive John of an active vacation. The morning of his flight home Cody called and said she wasn't feeling well; she was having trouble breathing.

"How much trouble, Cody? Shall I call an ambulance?"

"No, please, no. Just come over."

Cody was puffing her inhaler when Ernie and I got to her apartment. She didn't feel better. Her breathing was in short sips.

I said, "We need to go to the hospital, Cody."

She said, "Okay. But no ambulance. Let's just drive. John's coming, too."

Ernie drove. I kept my arm around Cody. Her breathing was in shallow gasps. I prayed for God to protect her. Cody's primary care doctor was affiliated with Fairview Southdale Hospital in the nearby suburb of Edina. I'd worked there for years before I was transferred to the Minneapolis hospital campus, so I knew some of the emergency room staff. As soon as I used the words "breathing distress" at the ER entrance, Cody was taken to an exam room. I followed and gave the nurse a copy of Cody's medical summary. In a flurry of activity, an oxygen mask was placed over her nose and mouth, and she was hooked up to monitors. The ER doctor ordered blood and urine tests, and chest x-rays.

"You can't do that," I told a clinician who was heading in the direction of Cody's urethra with a catheter to obtain a urine sample. "Cody has a Mitrofanoff; she can only be cathed through the bellybutton."

The clinicians all stopped and looked up at me. None of them had heard of a Mitrofanoff. The doctor asked what it was.

While the lab person drew blood, I explained the bladder augmentation surgery. Ernie joined us and demonstrated how catheterization was done. The clinicians seemed impressed with the surgical innovation. I was a little surprised that we knew more about it than they did.

Ernie said, "You can't use that," as the lab tech started to put a Band-Aid on Cody's arm. "It's latex." The lab tech paused. I suggested he use gauze and paper tape instead.

The doctor pointed to the blinking numbers on the screen overhead: 89, 90, 93. . . . "Those numbers need to stay above ninety. Cody's oxygen saturation was dangerously low—in the forties. Some people die before it gets that low. Next time something like this happens, don't hesitate to call an ambulance."

Yikes. Cody had been pale and limp in the car. I cringed realizing she could have *died!*

Ernie stayed with Cody while I went to the waiting room to tell John what was going on. He was attentive as I explained more about her medical situation. He knew a lot already from talking with Cody, but he had a few questions. His eyes were moving back and forth a little, which I took as an indication of his stress. He asked, "Has anything like this happened before?"

"No, this is new. She sometimes has asthma-like trouble with a cold, but nothing that ever put her in a hospital."

I went back to the exam room where Cody leaned partially upright on the gurney. She sobbed, "I don't want to scare John away by being sick."

I stroked her hair and said, "John is scared, sweetie. But I don't think you'll scare him away. He's scared because he cares about you."

Tears covered her cheeks as she said, "I want to see John."

I left to get him. I told John that Cody was afraid this would scare him away. He gave a firm "No" and followed me to the room. Cody gripped John's hand and he leaned close to her. Ernie and I waited outside for the test results.

Cody was diagnosed with pneumonia and "possible congestive heart failure." She was moved to the intensive care unit and put on IV antibiotics and diuretic medication. Lasix caused her to pee continually as fluid emptied from her lungs. She was too weak to cath herself. Paper tape held her catheter in place. A cannula with oxygen was put at her nostrils with tubing tucked behind her ears.

Before Ernie took John to the airport, Cody and John hugged and kissed, and she sobbed. He promised to call when he landed in San Francisco. I stayed with Cody.

She wept and blubbered again and again, "I miss John."

"Cody, you need to stop crying. This isn't helping you breathe. John wants you to get better."

She made a few more shudders and sobs before calming down.

Cody faced the standard complications in the hospital. There was a lot of explaining about the Mitrofanoff, reminders about latex, and the hospital had to special-order her catheters. I supervised her wound care. The skin on Cody's buttocks was in pretty good shape by then; I hoped to keep it that way. Her PCAs had still been placing protective bandages over delicate areas before pulling on her pants. I cautioned the nurses about the risk of skin breakdown but, inevitably, there was damage.

A pulmonologist ordered a BiPAP (bi-level positive airway pressure) machine to help Cody breathe while she slept. A facemask placed over her nose and mouth was connected with air hoses to the machine, which pumped air into Cody's lungs. A BiPAP was prescribed for her home use on a permanent basis.

The contraption took some getting used to. An air-moisturizing component was attached after a nosebleed. With the mask and hoses Cody looked like an alien, but she liked knowing she wouldn't stop breathing in her sleep. She admitted worrying about that since her apnea experience at fifteen.

For the five days Cody was in the hospital, John sent emails to my work again. He advised her to eat healthier, exercise, and ride around more in her wheelchair when she went home. He wrote, "I want to help you any way I can. Please don't get annoyed by my suggestions."

At a follow-up appointment, the pulmonologist suggested adding the new diagnosis of "respiratory failure" to Cody's medical summary. He was pleased that Cody was using her BiPAP and suggested an evaluation for sleep apnea. Since the treatment for sleep apnea was to use a BiPAP, and she already used one each night, the doctor didn't press her to be tested.

John visited again for three weeks in July and every two months thereafter. Each visit lasted two to four weeks and Cody burst into tears every time he left. John observed that Cody no longer snored now that she slept with the BiPAP. So he slept better, too.

When they weren't together, they were online for hours each day. If I called while they were "chatting" online, Cody included me in the conversation and told me again and again, "John is so sweet. I just love him."

The first time John came to our house for lunch, Cody warned me that he was uncomfortable around dogs. She gently lifted Dan onto John's lap to show him that the little dog, now old, was harmless. John gave Dan an awkward pat on the head. Blue put his front paws on John's lap but kept his greeting brief as though aware of John's reticence.

Our meal was in full swing when Blue quietly jumped on an empty chair and right up onto the dinner table—something he'd never done before. Stepping gingerly, he sat down in front of John's plate and stared at him. Cody and I exchanged eyebrow-raised smiles and glanced sideways at John, who sat between us.

Busy eating, John didn't notice the dog in front of him. Ernie saw Blue, but none of us moved or spoke. John finally looked up. Seeing Blue's snout a few inches in front of him, John said, "Well, hello."

Cody erupted in laughter. John and Blue were friends after that.

Cody's friend Gertrude cautioned, "Take it slow with John." She worried that he'd monopolize Cody's time. But Gertrude soon saw that Cody wanted her around whether or not John was there. Cody invited her to come with them to the Raspberry Festival in Hopkins, to street dances and outdoor concerts, restaurants, and out for ice cream. Gertrude joined in teasing John. Cody convinced him to try on girl's hats, and the three of them laughed. Cody went from teaser to defender, saying, "Aww, John, you look so adorable."

Gertrude was diagnosed with diabetes that summer. Cody worried about her friend. She stocked up on sugarless candy, diet drinks, and sugar-free Jell-O. If John or other visitors expressed interest in those snacks, Cody said, "Don't touch that. It's for Gertrude."

Cody squealed, "I love it when family comes!" My relatives were in town again for Christmas. Richard brought Mom and his fiancée, Dorene. His former wife, Fay, and daughter Joanna came, too. Despite a few divorces everyone remained friends. Cody appreciated that her family grew larger. She teased, "Uncle Richard, you're surrounded by all your women: your mother, your daughter, your sister, your niece, your former wife, and your future wife!"

John arrived two days after Christmas. Cody introduced him to the family. Mom kept calling him "Horky," the childhood nickname for my cousin Bill. I realized how much John actually resembled my cousin; they could have been brothers. Mom continued to call him "Horky." Cody gave up trying to correct her.

Cody noted a change in Mom that had become a growing concern for our family. "Grandma says the same things and tells the same stories over and over." Mom kept becoming anxious, thinking her purse was lost. Cody said again and again, "It's right here, Grandma. It's right where you left it."

As John left for California after this visit, Cody hugged him tight and tried not to cry. John said, "Don't worry. I'll be home again soon," now referring to "home" as Cody's place.

I was grateful for John's increasing presence in Cody's life, not only because he made her happy, but also for the peace of mind when Ernie and I made more frequent trips east to help my mother. Cody felt safer with John there when a new or substitute attendant came. She said the "good" PCAs liked John and joked around with him. Some "less good" PCAs did not appreciate his presence. She thought it was because John noticed if they didn't do their work.

Cody now researched sex for those with cerebral palsy. With the Internet she was far more successful than I'd been years before when I tried to find information on sex for women with physical disabilities. She looked up medical terms, conditions, and medications, and emailed me things she found interesting. While Cody learned more about CP, John wanted to know more about spina bifida. The four of us went to Rochester, Minnesota, for a Spina Bifida Association conference.

Much had been learned about the congenital neural tube birth defect since Cody was born. Although the cause was still unknown, a connection had been made to nutritional deficiencies of a B vitamin, folic acid, now a standard ingredient in prenatal supplements. Tests could be done early in pregnancy to determine whether a fetus had spina bifida. Stunning strides were being made in prenatal procedures to repair the defect or reduce the damage it caused. I was reminded that Cody was born at a time when surgical techniques and devices were advanced enough to save her life, but not enough to anticipate or prevent some related and ongoing health threats caused by spina bifida.

In the two years since Cody had become engaged, she often brought up wanting to meet John's parents. We tried to figure out how to make that happen. To go to California, she'd need to take a PCA. That meant two plane tickets, plus the cost of a PCA's time. John had to use crutches in his parents' home because it wasn't wheelchair accessible, which meant staying in a hotel in the Bay area, with an added room for the PCA. All that was more than we could afford.

Cody suggested that John invite his parents to the Twin Cities. Each time she brought up the subject, John gave a different reason why his parents couldn't visit. When she asked him direct questions about it, he suddenly had to go to the bathroom or retrieve his clothes from the dryer. When Cody pointed out that his series of excuses didn't make sense, John said the "real" reason was that his parents didn't like to travel. When he mentioned that his parents were vacationing with relatives in the Midwest, Cody confronted him. "I thought you told me your parents don't like to travel?" John became flustered and refused to discuss it further.

Cody was angry when she called to tell me about his deception. "He lied, Mom. And now he won't talk about it."

"Maybe he's embarrassed. Maybe his parents can't afford another vacation."

Cody asked, "You think that's it?"

"Well, you said they're retired. Traveling is expensive."

"But I really want to meet them."

I had an idea. "Tell John that Ernie and I are happy to buy airline tickets for his parents so they can come for a visit, and they're invited to stay with us."

"Cool! I'll tell him."

When he heard about our offer, John finally admitted the truth. He had not told his parents about his marriage proposal. Cody wanted an explanation.

John said he was afraid to tell his parents. He thought they'd disapprove of him marrying someone who lived so far from them; they might try to stop him from visiting Cody.

Cody spoke firmly to John. "How old are you? Four? Or forty? You're a grown man, John. You can say what's important to you. It's your life!"

She told him he should be proud of his decision and tell his parents the truth. But John said he couldn't. Cody was angry and said if he couldn't tell his parents about the engagement, then the engagement was off.

She told me, "He's never lived on his own, Mom. He depends on his parents for everything. I don't think he has the confidence to stand up for himself."

Cody and John now called their relationship a friendship. Both were free to date others. However, despite the official redefinition, nothing noticeably changed. John continued regular visits; Cody still cried when he left. When he was in town they cooked meals together and entertained as a couple. She continued to tell me how "sweet" John was and how much she loved him.

The day after Mother's Day, Ernie's mother died peacefully in her sleep. Cody cried when she heard the news and worried about Ernie: "Is he okay, Mom? He loved Grandma so much." Daily grief ambushed us all and delivered a follow-up punch two weeks later when our little dog Dan died of congestive heart failure. Cody cried that she didn't have a chance to say goodbye to her dog, but her grief was again tempered by concern for Ernie. She made a card professing her love, and spent Father's Day with him, as she now did each year.

Lorraine's death prompted me to think about wills. Mine needed an update, and Ernie and Cody didn't have wills. We named each other as executors, powers of attorney, and beneficiaries. John came along to the lawyer's office when we signed the documents in July. On the way home the four of us had a silly conversation about death. We joked and discussed the pros and cons of each one of us being the first to die. Was it better to live longer than our loved ones and be left alone? Or was it better to die sooner and have our loved ones with us to the end? Which would be harder? Which would be more painful for the other? We each changed our choices around a few times. The only thing we finally agreed upon was: we all wanted Ernie around until the end of our lives, because he was indispensable.

I remembered a similarly silly question I asked Cody when she was a teenager: "Would you rather be paralyzed and in a wheelchair all your life or be able to walk but be blind and deaf?" She had answered, "Neither one, Mom."

Chapter 25

Breathtaking

CODY TURNED TWENTY-SEVEN in August and wanted all her parents together for a birthday dinner at Michelangelo's, a restaurant where the waiters knew Cody and John by name. Dennis was now in love with a British woman and spent the summer in England. He and Penelope returned together, and Tad flew in from Philadelphia. Cody received a big welcome at Michelangelo's. The chef even came out to say, "Happy Birthday!"

Our waiter was a flamboyant fellow Cody hadn't met before. He saw she was a special guest and treated her as such. He teased me for ordering something that wasn't on the menu and noticed this entertained Cody. He embellished facial expressions and gestures and made friendly jokes at my expense throughout the meal. He brought big cups of coffee for everyone but served me a tiny demitasse cup. We were feeling merry and laughing together when he asked if we enjoyed our desserts.

Ernie winked at Cody and said, "Perhaps you'd like to meet Cody's parents."

Cody broke into a huge smile. Ernie gestured to me and said, "This is Cody's mother."

The waiter politely nodded as Ernie continued around the table. "This is Cody's original father. This is Cody's adoptive father." Looking back at the waiter he added, "And I am Cody's stepfather."

The waiter clasped his hands together, raised an eyebrow, and turned to me. "My, *my!* Haven't *we* been busy!" Cody burst out laughing.

Oscar had moved earlier that year to his tiny hometown of Menahga. Close in age, he'd been Cody's best friend in the building since she first moved there six years before. Now Oscar was John's friend, too. On a Saturday in September the four of us drove three hours north to visit Oscar. His two-room apartment was set up so that everything he used was within reach. The other residents in his building, all elderly, had similar needs for attendant help. There wasn't much to do in Menahga. Oscar rarely saw the few family members who lived nearby and seldom left his apartment. While we ate lunch, I asked Oscar why he moved to such a small town after living in the Twin Cities for so many years.

"In the Cities," Oscar said, "PCAs weren't there when I needed them. Here they are reliable." Oscar needed help with transfers to and from his wheelchair. When he had lived in Cody's building, PCAs left him on the toilet overnight more than once, without returning until morning. Some days, he was stuck in bed because his PCA didn't show up until the afternoon. Oscar missed his friends in the Twin Cities, but feeling safe was more important.

Dennis and Penelope married in October. Cody joined Penelope's parents and the pastors across the street for the small ceremony in Dennis's living room. Cody could not attend a larger celebration the next spring in England. Besides the expense and need for help with daily cares, long-distance travel was now too risky, with too much potential for a health emergency.

Only weeks later, Cody ended up in Fairview Southdale with respiratory distress again. This time, I called 9-1-1. I rode in the ambulance with her. Ernie followed in the car with John and her wheelchair. She was again diagnosed with pneumonia and given Lasix, oxygen, and IV antibiotics. John stayed overnight with Cody. I appreciated that as much as she did.

Recovery took five days and was measured by how little added oxygen Cody needed to maintain saturation in the 90s. I asked two experienced PCAs to be more available than usual (and hopefully more reliable) when Cody came home, because I would be unavailable to help out. I was having bunion surgery on both feet in early December.

Anticipating my operation gave me more perspective on Cody's bravery. I found it hard to ignore the dread that surfaced in the days before the surgery. Whenever I felt scared, I thought of her skill in focusing on positive thoughts and activities. She was so much better at it.

After surgery and one miserable night in the hospital, I was sent home with painkillers and told to keep my feet elevated for three weeks. On the fourth day, Ernie came home from work to find me tearful, miserable, and stir crazy. I felt sad and my feet throbbed. Pain medication probably exacerbated my melancholy. The phone rang; it was Cody. At the end of our chat, she said, "I wish I could wait on you, Mom." She sounded so sincere, tears spilled down my cheeks as I hung up.

Ernie asked, "Would you like to go see Cody?"

I blurted, "*Yes!*" before remembering that the farthest I'd gone in four days was to the bathroom. "Wait, I can hardly walk ten steps."

"We can do it. The spare wheelchair is in the garage. I'll lift you into the car if I have to."

I cried more as I thanked him. I wheeled to the car and Ernie steadied me as I slid into the front seat. With the seatback reclined I rested my gauze-wrapped feet on the dashboard. My mood lifted immensely, though I could see only the treetops and clouds against the winter sky.

Ernie had called ahead to tell Cody we were coming. She was waiting near the mailboxes in the lobby of her building. She wheeled in front of the automatic entrance and the glass door opened. I wheeled inside to see an expression on Cody's face that I'd never forget. Her eyes moved from my face to my hands on the wheels, to my bandaged feet on footrests, and back to my face, in silent recognition. I'd become a fellow tribe member.

"Hi, Mom."

"Hi, Cody."

She wheeled behind me as I guided my wheelchair around the corner to her apartment. I dropped my gloves as I went through the door.

Cody's voice sounded both consoling and excited as she asked, "Isn't it a drag when you drop something?" She handed me a reacher.

She kept three or four mechanical extenders in her apartment for picking up dropped items. The squeeze handles worked pretty well grabbing clothes, less well for paper or small objects. One had a magnet on the end.

My visit with Cody was charmed in a way I'd not experienced in her twenty-seven years. For a short time I was included in a different family with her. I was disabled, albeit temporarily, and Cody commiserated with my frustrations and inconveniences and helped me feel better.

John came after Christmas for almost a month. Five days before his flight back to California Cody developed severe breathing distress for a third time. Again she'd been especially active prior to the admission, again a urinary tract infection, and again her chart read "pneumonia and possible congestive heart failure." She was given the same tests and treatment.

Prior to discharge Cody put her mouth on the incentive spirometer to take deep breaths, but she could make the plastic ball rise only part way in short bursts. I asked her primary care doctor, "Why does this keep happening? What is wrong?" The doctor's expression remained impassive. He didn't look at me or answer before he left the room.

Cody scowled. "I don't trust that guy."

At a follow-up appointment with a pulmonologist, Cody was prescribed a nebulizer that changed liquid medicine to a mist inhaled through a plastic mouthpiece. A nebulizer helped her breathe in the hospital. Now she'd use one at home. The doctor didn't know the cause of her breathing problems but he suggested she be on oxygen—permanently. This meant using a nasal cannula and portable oxygen tank. Cody's face flushed as he spoke. With anger and firm conviction she said, "I don't want a plastic tube on my face. I'll look like a disabled person!"

I wanted to kiss her for not considering her wheelchair the more obvious tipoff. But this was serious; an expert had suggested a significant change to Cody's life.

I asked, "Are you saying it's *necessary* for Cody to be on oxygen at all times?"

The pulmonologist said, "I recommend it, but it's her choice. She has diminished lung capacity. At some point, she'll need oxygen 24/7."

Cody only heard, "It's her choice." The doctor had already looked away. He made no further argument to convince her.

I told Cody, "We can discuss this more at home before deciding."

Her eyes flashed as she said, "People on oxygen look like they're about to die!"

Cody remained adamant. Using oxygen on a permanent basis was tantamount to being a freak. I reminded her of others she knew who were on oxygen, but nothing I said mattered.

She vowed to address the problem by building strength and losing weight. The threat of being attached to an oxygen tank provided new motivation to exercise. Ernie and I took Cody to a sporting goods store and purchased two-, three-, and five-pound weights, and non-latex elastic bands for stretching. She found a workout video for people in wheelchairs. John suggested she take daily rides into downtown Hopkins—at least wheel to the corner and back.

Life returned to normal, meaning John came for a few weeks every two months. They enjoyed a busy social life. Cody's musician friend from Philly came to town several times. Cody brought John and other friends to see Pierce wherever his band played. Sometimes the musicians came back to Cody's, and they all talked late into the night.

Cody's friend Orlando wrote that he was moving back to the area. He'd been praying for Cody and looked forward to seeing her cross-stitch projects. Lewis had gone to California, but he and his mother, Cynthia, were now back in town. Cody arranged for all of them to meet John. Every friend of Cody's became a friend to John. His easygoing enjoyment of her affectionate teasing was fun to watch, as were his sweet ways of teasing her.

John often put his arm around Cody's shoulder and played with her hair. Sometimes he took a hairbrush from her backpack and swept hair away from her face while she focused on the computer or a cross-stitch project. The first time I saw him do that, Cody looked up with a matter-of-fact shrug of her shoulders and said, "He loves my hair."

As Cody's dependency on PCAs increased, so did the frequency of cancellations and no-shows. She had a constant fear of being stranded. After the umpteenth panicked morning call that she was stuck in bed with no PCA, I promised I would always help if a PCA didn't come. But I asked

Cody not to tell anyone about my promise. She could expect even more problems if PCAs knew a family member could help. Cody often heard, "You can get your mom, right?" or "Call your mother; she'll come."

As it was, my hospital job required full-time attention. Ernie had gone back to school for computer programming, and we were solely dependent upon my income. A staff of professionals reported to me, and I attended several meetings each week. I wasn't always able to leave my office to drive to Cody's apartment. I promised that she'd not be stuck, but we had to work around my schedule.

One day when Cody's PCA didn't show, I was in a mandatory morning meeting. Ernie went to help her. He had performed various cares for Cody before, but this was the first time he helped with her bowel emptying procedure. He put on a pair of vinyl gloves and asked her to tell him exactly what to do. He gagged and dry-heaved at every step, making continuous uncontrollable retching noises. Between gags, he said again and again, "I'm sorry; I'm sorry."

Cody laughed so hard her bowels emptied faster.

A few weeks prior to Cody's twenty-eighth birthday a giant box from Tad arrived at her apartment. Inside was a bi-directional cycle table. Electronic controls registered speed, distance, mileage, and cycle time. Adjustments allowed for variation in difficulty, and dials measured heart rate and calories burned. Cody could wheel forward under a platform and pedal the handles. She made an enthusiastic start with the machine and overdid it the first day. Despite instructions and reminders, she repeated this common mistake each time she began a new exercise regimen.

By the time Tad came on her birthday, Cody had strained muscles in her forearms and shoulders. Use of her arms was too essential to risk injury; she had to slow down. She created a schedule of activities for daily moderate exercise instead of spurts of frenetic motion. I don't know if she followed her schedule, because she refused to exercise with anyone watching.

Sandwiched between a mother, now diagnosed with Alzheimer's disease, and a daughter with so many complex physical and medical challenges, I began to consider my own mortality. My biggest fear was that my death would leave Cody without a rescuer. This worry became acute as her medical complications increased. I felt like the sole keeper of so much information about my daughter. Her physician specialists worked within three different hospital systems. She didn't have a single doctor who knew about all of her medical issues. Her primary care doctor had never met her urologist or her neurosurgeon, and so on. Tad was in Philadelphia and, with so much travel, Dennis was rarely around during her emergencies and no longer closely involved with Cody's healthcare. She had no siblings and none of my family lived in Minnesota. I knew Ernie would never abandon Cody. I could trust him to help her any way he could. But he was still in school.

I spoke to several lawyers. By September I signed an irrevocable trust for Cody. The trust was named beneficiary in Ernie's will and mine. By law, trust money was restricted from use for necessities such as housing. That way it would not compromise her disability benefits. However, it could be used for any extras to make Cody's life more comfortable. Even though Ernie and I were not wealthy, we could safely leave whatever we had to Cody. I felt some peace about this.

By Thanksgiving, the *fiancé* word was in use again. John wanted to move to Minnesota to be with Cody. She glowed. "I'm so happy; I'm just so happy. I can't wait. I love John."

Cody put John's name on the waiting list for an apartment in her building. I helped John fill out the application. To our surprise, a one-bedroom unit was available within two months.

Ernie and I picked up John at the airport on a Friday near the end of January. The caretaker gave John keys to his freshly painted apartment on the third floor. The moving truck was due in two weeks. I asked John how his family felt about his move. He said he hadn't actually told them about it until shortly before his flight. Until then, they assumed he was making his regular visit with Cody.

I asked, "Are you kidding? Why didn't you tell them before?"

John said he thought they'd try to talk him out of it. And his fears were well founded. His mother said relocation was "out of the question."

However, his parents talked privately and, though John never learned what was said, his mother told him his move to Minnesota was okay with her. In fact, Lois packed John's things for the moving truck, sending along everything she could think of that John might need.

Cody stayed home while I drove John to the Social Security Administration in Edina to transfer his disability benefits from California to Minnesota. We went then to the Department of Human Services office in Minneapolis to apply for medical assistance. He applied for a Minnesota ID at the driver's license bureau. I helped him fill out piles of forms for these things and agreed to be named as official helper on the multi-paged recertification forms that he was required to complete annually for any services. There was plenty of waiting involved with each step, but John was happy. He said it was an easier process than in California.

When the movers arrived, John was relieved that his valuables were unharmed. Even his video magnifier (that enlarged text) arrived safely. Cody was impressed with John's widescreen TV and immediately started saving to buy one for her apartment. John slept with Cody every night, so there was no rush to furnish his place. A friend who was moving offered a couch. Cody bought him two lamps with glass shades etched with his favorite images of timber wolves. He bought a platform bed, a card table for the kitchen, and two folding chairs to keep in the closet. Some items from Cody's apartment, and framed wild animal prints from a garage sale, finished the look.

John kept his apartment clean and clutter-free—a dramatic contrast to Cody's, where every surface was covered with crafts, papers, books, family photos, medical supplies, stuffed animals, dried flowers, plants, and knick-knacks. Her floor was clear for wheeling around and her kitchen was clean, but counters were covered with small appliances, recipe boxes, cookbooks, utensils, and baking accessories. Some of these went to their "upstairs" kitchen. Cody awoke every morning smiling. She hugged John and said, "I'm so glad you're here."

The couple's daily routine began when John unlocked the door for the morning attendant. He went to his apartment to shower and dress. He spent parts of every day upstairs, usually while Cody was with her PCA. They ate lunch together at either apartment, depending upon which cupboard or refrigerator was better stocked. John stayed in touch with family and friends by email and usually took an afternoon nap. Cody joined him upstairs to decide about dinner. Sometimes in the evening they each logged onto the Internet from their own apartments and joined each other and friends online for chatroom conversations.

Being together on a permanent basis had its adjustments. Cody sent an email in early February when Ernie and I were in Pittsburgh helping my mother. The word, "Stubborn" was written in the subject line:

Hi Mom and Ernie, Yes, I love having John with me, and I'm no longer lonely which is a good thing. However, why did I say I wanted him around all the time?? LOL Just kidding. You have absolutely no clue how annoyed I am. He just couldn't wait for someone to help him put together that damn vacuum cleaner he bought at Target the other day, so he tried to do it himself. He got frustrated, and when he gets uptight, he acts like Dad [Dennis] in one of his tirades. OH and NO MOM, I am not like that anymore myself. I TRIED to tell him to wait before he bought the stupid thing in the first place, but he didn't listen. He does his own thing. I'm just not going to get caught up in his childishness. I leave whichever apartment we're in at the moment of his obnoxiousness, and go to the other one. I LOVE having him around MOST of the time. The reason I am sooooooo MAD: He absolutely, positively wanted this vacuum up and running, and just wanted it so bad, that I got a friend to help put it together except for one missing tiny screw. I went to my apartment for ten minutes, and when I got back, the #@%# had the thing in pieces again. If I didn't love him, I'd smack him a good one right now. We spent the whole fricken morning figuring out the stupid thing. He can't get it back together, so he went to the hardware store to get packing tape, and called Metro to get a ride to take it back to Target tomorrow. I didn't call him a big pain in the ass to his face, but I thought that. He loses his keys daily due to his eyesight, and has a tirade because he feels so stupid at the time. Sometimes it's like living with Dad again with the exception that, with John, I feel free to say, "Shut the h___ up," and he does—MOST of the time. Earlier I thought about a wish I had once. I wished I had a man with a baby that I could adopt like Dad did with me, and I think God heard that, and got mixed up and thought I said, "I want a man who acts like a baby." I'm not sure I want a man at the moment. LOL. But, I'm not lonely, and he's sweet half of the time, and he does take care of me when he is not stressed out, which is a big plus. There is another good thing—when he is stressed, it forces me to think better, and be the adult, which is good for my self-esteem. Do you have any advice for me with John? I put him on a TIME OUT for the moment. I've also stopped giving him advice. I'm letting him make his own mistakes. I'm sure if I ignore him long enough, he'll come to his senses, and see how dumb he behaved. I hope you are having better luck with Grandma. Give her a kiss for me. I love you. Cody

She provided an update the following day:

Hi Mom, I just wanted to say that things are going better today. John's behaving. Heehee. I talked to his mom about his fits. She called him and told him to "Knock it off and listen to Cody." LOL. I called her because he was acting so obnoxious, and I wondered if he threw fits at home. Apparently he has, and she doesn't like it either. Then she sent me a very sweet email and said, "I'm glad you're patient with him, and you're doing very well with him. He seems to be very happy. I'm glad that he's there." Well. Talk to you tomorrow. Oh yeah, can Ernie come over on Tuesday and fix the toilet again please? I think it needs a whole new mechanism in it. I'm having trouble with [the caretaker]. Cody

The same week, Cody had tickets to see one of her favorite boy bands, NSYNC. None of her girlfriends could go so she begged John to come with her to the concert. His musical taste was more in line with hard rock, but he was a good sport. "You should have seen John in the middle of all the screaming girls!" Cody laughed heartily adding, "He was so cute!"

Cody and John took frequent bus rides to Target or Michael's craft store. John went next door to look at electronics while Cody spent hours looking at threads and beads.

A Metro Mobility dispatcher put Cody back in touch with her friend Rachel. Rachel had lived for two years in an assisted-living facility after high school. The program was designed to foster independence, but Rachel found it restrictive. She was discouraged from going out without an able-bodied companion. At the time, Cody had been fairly vocal with Rachel about how discriminatory and unfair that was. When Rachel moved to an even more controlled residence, she remained out of contact with Cody for several years. The day a Metro dispatcher mentioned Cody by name, Rachel asked for her phone number. She told Cody, "I felt like a lost cause. I was ashamed to tell you where I lived. I knew you would be appalled. But I missed you. You always cheered me on." Cody had missed Rachel, too. From then on, Cody, Rachel, and John were together often.

Cody corresponded with Student Support Services at Hennepin Technical College about finishing her associate degree. She'd left Normandale Community College before taking math courses. Placement tests were the next step. Instead of more tests Cody opted to use the Internet to learn about things that interested her. She wanted to know how her brain worked, how it was different than she thought it should be, especially after neurosurgeries when she noticed some memory loss or a tendency to drop things. She wanted to know why it was hard to read for any length of time, why she was easily distracted or daydreamed so much.

Cody could assemble complicated mechanical things, computer parts, stereos, and complex remote control devices—things I couldn't figure out, or remember how to do, even if given careful instruction. I once handed her a multifunctional clock with several unlabeled buttons that I'd fiddled with to the point of exasperation. Even Ernie didn't know how it worked. Cody tinkered with the clock for less than a minute before successfully setting the time. She never read instructions; she just figured things out.

She found a test for attention deficit disorder (ADD) listing forty questions. The more yeses you answered, the more likely you had ADD. Cody answered yes to all but one question. She was pretty excited to have identified a condition to explain various difficulties she'd experienced in her thinking and learning. Shortly before John left to visit his parents in April, Cody emailed me an article that said people with ADD could be good creative writers. I thought of the stories Cody wrote in school. Her tales were entertaining, imaginative, and still funny after so many years.

I emailed back:

> I was struck by the part about people with ADD being good creative
> writers. You've always been a good writer. Maybe writing is something
> you could do that could also make money. You could write articles about
> things you think about. I could help as an editor. I believe you're good
> enough to be published. You wrote good journals and short stories in
> school, and you're very good at describing things. Plus, you have a good
> vocabulary. Think about it. I love you.

Cody responded:

> I have thought about the writing thing, and thought I'd write a bio about
> my life, but everyone does that. It's boring. I have been thinking about
> it actually, and thought it might be fun writing children's books. For
> one, it's at my level of ability and interest. I am not sure about this, but
> was thinking about writing a book about my life, but who wants to read
> about some woman who had a bunch of surgeries and junk? It's already
> been done, and those people always come across to me as if they are
> trying to make people feel sorry for them. I know they are just trying to
> make people aware. But the books I read like that sound like the people
> are just whining about their hardships, instead of how interesting living
> a life having to use a wheelchair can be. How the struggles of life may
> look horrible to the "normal person"—but to us, we are just living—like
> them. Well, okay, maybe a couple people have had good books like that,
> but who wants to hear about more things like that? I'd need to convince
> myself that there would be someone interested before making myself do
> it. It would be a lot of hard work for me. I told John what you said, and he
> went crazy, "Yeah, yeah, yeah. You should do it Cody. Do it. You're a great
> speaker." I think he meant writer or thinker. Maybe I will. John's leaving in
> a few days, and I'm not bawling my eyes out. That's a switch. LOL.

Cody told me, "I'm worried John won't come back once he's home with
his parents."

"Why do you think that? You're both happy. He loves having his own
place."

With a smirk she said, "Well, he didn't tell his parents when he decided to move here." I laughed, and she added, "I don't think he'd really do that, but it kept coming into my head."

"You better talk to John about your worries."

She did, and John said, "Cody, of course I'm coming back. We're together now. That's it. Now I live here with you. But I still want to see my family a couple times a year."

When she told him she was afraid he'd call from California and tell her to sell his stuff because he wasn't coming back, John scoffed. "You just find things to worry about." He patted her shoulder and said, "Relax, I'm coming back, you silly goose."

Cody felt better after the talk. But I think she held onto a tiny doubt until he returned that first time.

Chapter 26

Cousins

DESPITE EXERCISE and small meals, Cody hadn't lost a single pound. She was frustrated. My own concern must have been over the top, based on her email in April 2001. Cody often broached serious topics in writing, so she could make her entire point without being interrupted.

Hi Mom, In order for me to keep losing weight, there are a couple of things that you and a couple of others need to stop doing in order to help me. First, if I decide to go out to eat or you see something to eat in my home that is unhealthy, stay out of it, and don't question it. It is my life, and my body. Yes, sometimes I eat the wrong stuff. I know that. I have enough self-frustration without others adding to it. I want to lose weight, but it is harder on me if I have someone constantly asking me about the things I eat. That is not healthy or helpful for me. Plus, I act as though I am not listening, when I am really just feeling bad. It may seem like a helpful thing to you, and I know you are concerned. It's just hard when people—not just you—tell me things like, "Oh you shouldn't eat that if you want to lose weight," or, "Boy that has a lot of calories in it." I know the things that are bad for me, and, yes, reminders are good, but not constant ones. So, together we can figure out how to help me without making me feel self-conscious about what I eat. I have been eating healthier in the past week. When John came back, he saw me eating salads and oranges, and he said, "Cody, did we decide to eat healthy? That's good." I will bring some oranges for lunch tomorrow. I just counted the days, and if I really stick to it, I could be down to 100 pounds by the Fourth of July. John said he's going to help me too. See ya. Cody

I promised to stop mentioning Cody's weight. She asked me to tell Dennis to stop his reminders, too. I found it hard to let go of the worry though. I could see that moving around and maintaining the independence she valued were becoming more difficult.

While Ernie and I were in Pittsburgh with Mom in early May, Cody sent an email about an all-day effort to find a PCA in the face of consecutive cancellations. Her lone choice was a young woman who'd help only if she could bring her child. The active toddler tore up Cody's apartment and "wracked John's nerves." Cody ended her note saying she "sure could use some words of encouragement."

I responded: "Here are some words of encouragement: You are smart, clever, creative, and we are both very proud of you. You are a great problem-solver, and you are sweet, and funny, and cute, too. Love, Mom"

She emailed back that night:

> Funny, Mother. Thanks for the words of encouragement. Today was a very long day, but on the upside, John looked really cute talking with the little kid. The kid wracked his nerves again, but it was cute to watch. I'm so glad I'm not having kids. John wants to learn how to take care of my wounds, so we never have another day like today. One more thing—Happy Mother's Day. I love you.

An ambulance took Cody to Fairview Southdale Hospital in late May, again in June and in August. The same breathing problems and symptoms were attributed to pneumonia and possible congestive heart failure. The May emergency coincided with a metro-wide nursing contract dispute that included issues such as safe staffing levels. National media attention focused on Twin Cities hospitals as negotiations were underway to avert a strike.

Cody had worn the bright yellow "I Support Minnesota Nurses" T-shirts in 1984 when 6,000 nurses were on strike in the Twin Cities. Even as a child Cody knew she depended on nurses more often than most. Nurses could make the difference between a safe hospital experience and a miserable one—in some cases between life and death.

We saw no obvious stress associated with the escalating dispute as

Cody was tested, x-rayed, and treated again with IV antibiotics, Lasix, and oxygen. But once Cody was moved from the ICU to the sixth floor, mishaps occurred throughout her stay that we assumed were the result of nurses' stress.

I provided extra copies of Cody's one-page medical summary. A nurse suggested I write the food allergy list on the dry-erase board next to the bed. Despite precautions, meal trays consistently included items on Cody's allergy list. I warned her to be careful. More than one nurse told Cody, "I haven't had time to look at your chart."

When Cody pressed the call button it was sometimes up to forty minutes before anyone came . . . *if* anyone came. We struggled to find ways to convey and receive information about her care. Nurses were too busy to treat Cody's wounds, so I came each morning and evening to change dressings. I had to ask for bandages and catheters many times. I finally left the hospital to find a medical supply store to buy antibiotic ointment and latex-free catheters that had not been ordered in time. On the third day, a nurse told us that Cody's buttocks wounds were not even noted in her chart.

I arrived one day as Cody ate lunch. She appeared to move in slow motion due to her low oxygen saturation. As she lifted a forkful of dessert to her mouth, I shouted, "Cody, stop! It's peaches!" She dropped the fork with a start and made the "yikes" face. She had almost eaten something that would close her throat and cause her face to swell.

I was no longer comfortable leaving Cody alone in the hospital. I recalled the ER doctor's warning years before. *Hospitals are dangerous places.*

John spent each night with Cody. Ernie and I alternated being with her during the day when John went home to shower or nap. Her primary care doctor was on vacation. His associate was more forthcoming with information and noticeable concern. He admitted being puzzled by her ongoing respiratory problems.

Cody's June hospitalization departed from all previous experience. She was admitted toward the end of a twenty-three-day nurses' strike. Replacement nurses had been brought in from other states.

In the ambulance Cody worried, "I won't know any of the nurses."

John, Ernie, and I vowed to be extra vigilant and not leave her alone.

A charge nurse on the sixth floor greeted Cody and introduced himself. He told her to let him know if she needed anything or had questions during her stay. Each day she was told what to expect concerning tests, nursing care, and mealtimes. There was immediate communication about physician visits, test results, and medications. A nurse inspected the meal trays to make sure nothing was served that Cody was allergic to. When a tray came with food on Cody's list, the charge nurse immediately called dietary services to correct it. We continued to worry about the lack of progress in discovering why Cody kept getting so sick. But the excellent communication and continuity of her care during the strike brought down our stress a notch.

On the day of Cody's discharge, the strike had just ended. Cody helped write an email to a hospital administrator describing her differing care before and during the strike. She stressed how communication was crucial for a frightened hospital patient. An email response the next day expressed thanks for sharing "important information" and included an apology. Process and service improvements were being identified and specific follow-up was occurring "as a result of" her feedback. I called Cody to read the email to her as she recuperated at home. I could hear her smile. She was pleased and impressed that information about her experience was helpful.

Ernie and I went to Cody's apartment every night for the next few days. The new evening PCA was not adept at securing bandages. The morning PCA reported finding the wounds uncovered and wads of gauze bunched up in Cody's pants. While I readjusted bandages and showed the PCA how to secure the gauze without putting tape on delicate skin, Ernie noticed that a medication Cody was supposed to be taking was still in the pill container. She'd forgotten the midday antibiotic. He asked her about that and also if she remembered to take her zinc pill.

Cody stammered, "Yes, I took it today."

Ernie frowned but didn't say anything more about the pills. He looked in her backpack and frowned again. "Where are the medical summary copies we brought the other day?"

Cody said, "They're here. I forgot to put them in the bag." She began to look annoyed as the PCA and I shuffled through papers on the desk. "I'll find them when you guys leave."

In the car Ernie said, "She was lying; she didn't take her zinc."

Cody called me at work the next morning. "What is up Ernie's butt?"

"He was mad that you weren't more careful taking your pills. And the summaries weren't in your backpack. If you had an emergency in the night, you wouldn't be prepared."

"If that bothered him so much, why didn't he say so?"

"I think he would have if your PCA wasn't there."

That afternoon, I received an email at work.

Hi Mom, I've been thinking about your telling me that Ernie was mad at me. First of all, why would you tell me instead of him telling me? That's not very nice. He should have told me himself, no matter who was there. If something's on our minds—we just say it. Isn't that what you've always taught me? Ernie's been acting nasty the past few nights, but I couldn't figure out why, because I've not done a thing that I know of. Granted, I do agree that I need some improving, but I happen to be doing quite well remembering ALL my medicine this time, and actually it's a challenge for me. It's hard to remember the pill in the middle of the day. I'm kind of proud of myself for going this long without a slip up. So if I slip with a few vitamins here and there, I don't see it as a crime. I've been doing okay no matter what Ernie says. I'm very hurt—he can speak for himself, or get over it. Oh, and those medical sheets—I took them out to clean my backpack. I felt bad that I forgot to put them back, but they are there now. Cody

I wrote back:

Hi Babe, You are right that Ernie should tell you himself if he's mad about something. As I told you, he meant to tell you right away, but we haven't seen you in private since you came home from the hospital. Neither of us would bring up such topics in front of others. I'm sure he will talk to you when he has the chance. I believe he considers it too important to discuss on the phone. I agree he was a bit nasty last night about the zinc, and he owes you an apology. He's been crabby for a few days with a headache and stress—which is no excuse for being nasty—however he was very worried about you. He gets upset when you're sick, and he is more sensitive than the average guy. He's also concerned about Ryan [Ernie's eight-year-old nephew]. We just found out Wednesday night that he has diabetes. Mark and Julie are heartbroken. We visited them yesterday in the hospital. Little Eric has been upset about it—crying. Ryan seems to be the only one who's fine. He's not bent out of shape at all. But in some ways he's too young to realize what it means to have a serious disease. I don't think Ernie was mad that you missed a pill. He gets mad—as I do—when he thinks you aren't being honest. That's the down side of occasionally lying to parents; we sometimes can't tell when you are telling the truth. If you're not sure if you took a pill, just say you're not sure. Trust is important in every relationship. I am very proud of you, and the energy you're putting into your healthcare. I love you. See you later. Mom

Cody's response was only about her young cousin.

Mom, Oh no . . . is there anything I can do? Can I go to visit baby Ryan? I love that kid, and I miss him, and the others. Actually I miss Ernie's whole family. We need to do something. That's just awful. Ryan's the little one, right? Yeah, Eric's the funny older one who reminds me of Zach when he was that age. Now I see why Ernie's been stressed the last few nights. Ask the family if they want me to come and sit with Ryan. He's a child, and he shouldn't be left alone and scared. The family needs a break from time to time. Poor Uncle Mark and Julie. (Am I supposed to know?) Uncle Mark is so sensitive. He's probably just devastated. That's so sad. How can a kid get that anyway? Cody

Another email followed immediately.

Subject: I've been meaning to say thank you.
Mom, I realize you guys really worry about me, and I just wanted you to know that I really appreciate all that you do for me. I do wish there was something special besides my taking better care of myself that I could do for you in return. I understand that taking care of me and basically having me is a struggle, and you do really well. I'm proud to say you're my mom

and Ernie's cool too—even if he doesn't handle his frustrations well. I know it is because he cares so much and feels helpless at times when he thinks I'm not thinking for myself. Have more faith in me—I'm not that bad. Remember, I could be worse, like [a friend] who is not as fortunate to have parents like you. I shudder to think. Talk to you later. Cody.

I answered:

Dear Cody, You are very welcome. You don't realize that taking care of yourself is the best and most wonderful gift I could ever get from you. That is the only really important thing I worry about. Caring for you is not a struggle—you are a bit high-maintenance at times—but most things of high value come at a high price. And you aren't too high-priced for me. You are wonderful, and I have great faith in you. You are a great addition to the world, and I am very glad you are here. You are right about Ernie with each thing you said. See you later. I love you! Mom

To offset continuing problems with PCAs, John was determined to learn how to help with Cody's personal cares. His vision impairment precluded his evaluating the wound healing or skin condition, but he wore the vinyl gloves and was now able to do most things she needed whenever necessary. John's help was invaluable to me especially during the month of July, when I had to focus on other family emergencies.

Finding a safe residence for my mother had become a priority in recent months. She continued to deny memory problems despite her diagnosis of "moderate to severe" Alzheimer's. A private-care home with six memory-impaired people in the suburb of Minnetonka had an opening in July. But we needed an effective strategy to gain Mom's cooperation in the move.

I told her about a friendly "bed and breakfast" with all meals and comforts included. I emphasized the nearness to Cody and John, and also to Ernie and me. Mom said she'd think about it. Ernie and I planned a drive to Pittsburgh to pick up a truckload of Mom's things. Charlie and his wife Edie would fly with Mom to Minnesota. Two terrible things happened before our plan could be accomplished.

Blue's health deteriorated suddenly due to advanced prostate cancer.

Our poor dog peed blood and became weak. A new medication helped Blue rally, but then Ernie almost died of kidney failure from a severe food poisoning. He spent three days in the hospital and was still wobbly a week later, but he didn't want to disrupt our plans for Mom's move.

Cody and John were worried. "He can stay at my place; I'll sleep at John's. I'll wait on Ernie hand and wheels. John and I will take care of him. We don't want to see anything worse happen to Ernie. You guys wouldn't want me to do that sort of thing so soon after a life-threatening experience, right?"

Ernie thanked Cody sincerely and assured her he was well enough.

When John said he was worried that he wouldn't know what to do if Cody became sick while we were gone, I gave him a list of contact numbers and put copies of her updated medical summary in her backpack and taped some to her wall–within sight and reach. I assured John, "If there's a problem, all you need to remember is: call an ambulance and take the medical summary along to the hospital. Then call us. We'll drive straight back."

A friend stayed with Blue while we were gone and Mom's move went smoothly. When she saw her new place she noticed her paintings on the walls, her clothes in the closet, and family photos with her Bible on the dresser. She looked around the room and announced, "I'll take it!"

We didn't see Mom for a week in early August during Cody's next breathing emergency. The doctor on call ordered new tests and explained a result that showed a high carbon dioxide level in Cody's blood. She was not absorbing adequate oxygen. He suggested adding "She hypoventilates" to Cody's medical summary to describe this condition.

This particular hospitalization represented a turning point in my thinking about Cody's recent health challenges. The shift occurred when I caught myself scolding her for not calling me when a doctor came to see her. I was angry to have missed a chance to ask questions or learn new diagnostic information.

Cody's voice sounded weak when she said, "I'm sorry, Mom; I forgot." A stab of guilt struck me for being so heavy-handed with her. Her low oxygen made it a challenge for her to think straight in the first place, let alone remember my instructions. I pushed her to exercise, eat right, take her pills, and be responsible. She was brave; she worked hard to be healthy. She never gave up, never lost her fire, and never held it against me when I came on so strong. I needed to tell her that, and apologize.

I told Cody how truly sorry I was. "You know, babe, this illness isn't your fault. You didn't do anything wrong to make yourself sick. Something is going on that we don't understand, but you're doing a good job. Nor is this happening because of something you didn't do. It isn't because you made a mistake."

Like every interchange with Cody wherein I expressed regret for some misdeed in my mothering, Cody responded with some version of "It's okay, Mom. It's no big deal."

Cody spoke to Julie and Zach by phone as usual from her hospital bed. They prayed together when she was scared. Zach sang songs to entertain her. The cousins made plans to see each other in a couple of weeks for Cody's twenty-ninth birthday. Julie's fiancé, Geoff, was also coming to meet Cody and John. Cody was ecstatic with anticipation and determined not to let her health interfere with their fun. She felt weak, became winded easily, and continued to gain weight. But it was birthday season and seeing her cousins was *almost* the only thing on her mind.

Subject: Worried about Grandma and had a thought
Good morning Mom, I had a vision in my sleep last night, and it made me come up with an idea for us. I'm worried about this whole Grandma thing. I don't want you to overwork yourself. You have a highly stressful job now, and Grandma is high maintenance. You can't do all that alone. I know you have Ernie, but he's sick, and can't do a lot for you right now. I feel helpless because her place doesn't have an elevator yet. Grandma needs more familiar faces around her. She may not remember John as John, but she seems to think he is another relative. So I suggest that in order to give you breaks, and for Grandma to still have family around, I could persuade John to visit her every so often. He's easy to get to do things. First of all, he's concerned about Grandma, and secondly, he's like a beagle. Someone just has to give him food, like maybe a sandwich

at Quizno's, and he'll do just about anything you ask him to. LOL. Just kidding. Anyway, John has an ability I don't. He can get up any hill. He can also climb stairs in his chair. That's something you may not know. At least I've seen him do it. Plus, he said if there's a fire, he could get out. So what I'm saying is, I can ask John to spend time with her, since I can't get in myself. What do you think? It's not me, but it's as close as we're going to get without you or Ernie going there. You can't take on all that by yourself, at least I'd rather you didn't. Talk to you soon. Cody.

I thanked Cody for her thoughtfulness and laughed at the reference to John as beagle-like. She often said he had all the best qualities of a dog. That was high praise.

Julie and Zach brought taped music they wrote for Cody. Their song had rhyming verses with cousin-loving lyrics, choruses of "*Whoa, whoa, whoa*" and an instrumental background. Their visit was filled with high-energy activities and nonstop laughter. John and Zach were Cody's two favorite people to tease, and she had them together. She cajoled them to sing a duet. John was not a singer; their duet sounded awful. Cody's facial expressions made Zachary laugh.

Julie's fiancé worked as a pharmaceutical rep for a drug company. Cody was very pleased to know an "inside" person who could explain things about prescription medicine. Geoff was also a cardio-pulmonary physiologist. He showed Cody how to use her exercise cycle more effectively. He explained it in a way that inspired Cody to exercise without overdoing it.

"Do almost nothing at first. Start with the tiniest movement, and do that for two weeks. Then add the slightest greater movement, and do that for two weeks. Add just a little tiny bit each time. You'll slowly build up your endurance. Play your favorite music at the same time."

Cody liked the idea of starting with almost no activity, and the part about doing it to music was especially appealing. "I can do that!"

The group wandered around town. Julie drove when they went by car. John was the navigator. Cody had no sense of direction. By now family lore was that the "blind guy" was the one who knew best how to get anywhere. John also led the way at the State Fair. They munched fried pickles and posed for a group picture printed on T-shirts. The cousins took turns pushing Cody when she became tired. Zach whizzed Cody around ramps in the animal barns.

When it was Julie's turn to push, she pointed out "hot guys" and at times "accidentally" wheeled into them. Cody said she'd used that technique to meet cute guys in high school. She'd roll over a boy's toe or bang into his knees and say she was so sorry.

Julie said, "Hot guy at three o'clock." Cody looked, became embarrassed and laughed. John good-naturedly endured Cody's observations about cute guys the same way he tolerated her crushes on singers in boy bands.

Julie noticed that John paid close attention to Cody's personal needs. He reminded her to put on sunscreen and, when it was time for her to get cathed, guided her to the First Aid Station where there were accommodations for her privacy. Once alone, Julie asked Cody about John's character and what she loved about him.

Cody said, "John is so sweet. He encourages me. He told me I am the most beautiful woman in the world."

Julie responded, "Aww, really? That's so sweet."

Cody smiled and joked, "Julie. You know he's legally blind . . ."

On the final day of the visit Ernie and I had a birthday gathering for Cody at our house. She arrived with a bag of laundry tied with ribbons and a card that read, "To Mother Who gave birth to me 29 years ago. Here is a gift to show you can still help with my laundry. I love you. Love, Cody." She closed her eyes and scrunched her shoulders as I kissed her twenty-nine times on her cheeks, forehead, eyelids, and chin.

At the end of three days of Cody's favorite types of fun with her cousins, they told each other "I love you" and "It's been a blast." Cody cried saying goodbye.

John's parents, Lois and Rich, came to stay in John's apartment for a week in September. The six of us met for dinner at Michelangelo's. Lois and Rich were sweet people who seemed shy in contrast to most of Cody's family. We made small talk to get to know each other. Rich's eyes twinkled as he described the first phone call from Cody four years before. He had called John to the phone saying, "It's a girl."

Rich had been startled and amused when Cody snapped back, "I'm not a girl. I'm a woman!" He and Cody now exchanged affectionate smiles.

Lois was a retired nurse who spent hours in libraries and town halls researching family history. She was especially interested in an ancestor who fought in the American Revolution. She said the name of the small town he was from in western Pennsylvania.

Surprised, I said, "That's next to the little town where my mother was born!"

Lois mentioned the name of her ancestor and Ernie looked up quickly. He'd seen my mother's Daughters of the American Revolution papers on our last trip to Pittsburgh. The same name, William Bloom, was listed in our family records. My grandfather was a direct descendent of a soldier by that name who served with George Washington at Valley Forge. Ernie asked Lois, "Do you know the birth date of your William Bloom?"

Lois gave the date, and it was the same birth date as my ancestor. Cody's eyes lit up. She said to John, "We're kissing cousins!"

Lois later asked me about Cody's health. I told her about the breathing problems and recent hospitalizations. She expressed heartfelt concern for Cody; she could see John loved her very much. We shared "mother happiness" that our kids each had someone special to love.

Ernie and I stopped by John's apartment to say goodbye to his parents the night before their flight home. We hugged and I told Lois and Rich how neat it was to have found our family connection. We wished them a safe trip back to California.

But the following morning their flight was cancelled. Hijacked airplanes had flown into the World Trade Center and the Pentagon. Another plane crashed in western Pennsylvania. All commercial airplanes were grounded. The TV endlessly replayed footage of the devastating explosions and described the horror and tragic aftermath. Our family joined millions of others calling relatives and friends around the country to make sure our loved ones were safe.

Chapter 27

Sweet Conversations

WHILE THE COUNTRY mourned the events of 9/11, Cody's health declined at an alarming rate. An EKG confirmed pulmonary hypertension and mild congestive heart failure. Her doctor prescribed a small daily dose of Lasix, but she was bloated, nauseous, and had a sharp pain in her left side when Ernie and I took her to the ER at the University of Minnesota Hospital campus of Fairview. ER physicians decided Cody didn't need to be admitted, but she needed to see a cardiologist right away.

The cardiologist prescribed heart medication, a higher dosage of Lasix, and oxygen—24/7. Cody firmly stated that she didn't want to be on oxygen. Her voice quivered as she gave her reasons. The doctor gently explained that Cody could become sicker without it.

I felt desperate, trying to convince her to take the doctor's advice. But Cody refused. Within two weeks she was much, much sicker.

Cody was admitted to the cardiac unit at the University Hospital, and for the next few days I feared for her life. She was surrounded with experts and activity as she underwent an aggressive series of diagnostic tests and treatments. Cody struggled to breathe when she lay down. Unable to balance herself or change position on the air mattress, she felt trapped and opted to sleep sitting in her wheelchair next to the hospital bed, wrapped in blankets, with a sheet pulled over her head (to "feel safer"). The next nurse to come into her room jumped and made a little squeal. Cody peeked out from under the sheet. The startled nurse exhaled and said, "I thought you were dead!" Cody had a good laugh.

John, Ernie, and I alternated nights on a cot in her room. Dennis visited sometimes during the day. My office was a brief shuttle ride to the other side of the Mississippi River, so I visited Cody at lunchtime and changed her dressings each morning and evening. I could tell the nurses appreciated that by how readily bandage supplies were brought to me. Various specialists came in each day, including Dr. Lee, her urologist from Gillette, who was also affiliated with University Hospital. Cody spoke by phone to Tad, Zach, Julie, and Charlie, and asked Geoff about any new medicines she was given.

The three-and-one-half-year nightmare with her breathing was finally addressed; high doses of diuretics produced dramatic results. It took a week, and some of it was grisly. I tried not to watch while clinicians put a peripherally inserted central catheter (PICC) in her arm. The PICC line made it easier over a prolonged period to administer IV medication and access blood without so many needle pokes. I looked into Cody's eyes, but in my peripheral vision I saw blood drip onto the sheets.

During my nights with Cody we had the sweet conversations that accompanied her all-too-frequent near-death experiences. She pointed out which residents she thought were cute. We said prayers, whispered about our fears, and made jokes about what was happening. She held my hand to fall asleep.

In a matter of days, Cody peed away an astonishing forty pounds of water weight. Her ankles and feet were no longer swollen; she could sit and lie down comfortably. She was relieved to realize it wasn't her diet or overeating that had caused her progressive weight gain. The fluid retention was also blamed for the worsening pressure sores on her buttocks. A wound care physician explained that pressure had been coming from the *inside*. The severe pressure sores could now begin to heal.

Cody came home from the hospital with a new pile of medications and under the care of a new team of physicians. Impressed with the comprehensive attention she received at the University Hospital, we found a University Clinic primary care doctor in the same building as her urologist, new pulmonologist, cardiologist, and—with the retirement of her neurosurgeon in St. Paul—a new neurosurgeon.

"Restrictive lung disease" was now the first diagnosis listed on Cody's medical summary. Her pulmonologist did not speak gently when he told Cody that she *must* be on oxygen 24/7. She had *no choice*. The cardiologist explained that the right ventricle in Cody's heart did not work as well as it should. A blood thinner was prescribed to prevent embolisms in the heart or lungs. The dosage often needed adjustment. If it was too high, Cody bruised easily or had blood in her urine.

John, Ernie, and I all went with Cody to her doctors' appointments. Physicians and nurses usually looked surprised the first time they saw us crowd into the exam room. Cody and John backed in their wheelchairs like cars in a small parking lot. We asked about medications and treatments. It was helpful to have more than one person hear what doctors advised.

Using oxygen 24/7 was the most difficult lifestyle change. Portable tanks in two sizes were delivered to Cody's apartment. An electric oxygen concentrator sat by her bedroom door for use while she slept. A cannula was attached to long tubing from the machine so she could also move around the apartment. Cody didn't mind using it while she slept, but she didn't want to be seen in public with oxygen. The topic inspired many arguments.

Two pressure sores from Cody's long hospital stay required more complicated care. Not all PCAs were comfortable dressing the "stage 3" wounds in the deeper layers of tissue. Infection and penetration to the bone were the threats to avoid. I went to the apartment every night and many mornings before work to change bandages and show new PCAs how.

The severity of the wounds prevented Cody from attending Julie and Geoff's wedding in St. Louis. However, she stayed in regular contact with each of them and, of course, Zach. She had questions for Geoff about how to strengthen her breathing and stimulate her heart so she wouldn't need medication or oxygen. She did online research, read material the pharmacy provided with each new prescription, and asked Geoff if medications were safe. She asked what the idea behind the drug was, what the benefits were, and what he thought the doctor would do to counteract a bad reaction or side effect.

She asked things like, "Am I gonna end up with liver cancer? Is it gonna kill me?" or "Why would taking water out of my body make me dizzy?" She asked friends who took the same drugs which side effects they experienced. She compared dosages and checked brand names with generic names to make sure she had the right pills. Sometimes she called Geoff with questions on behalf of her Internet friends.

Geoff took Cody's questions seriously and pulled out his medical books and *Physicians' Desk Reference*. He did his best to reassure her, and regularly reminded her that he wasn't a doctor. He suggested she ask her doctor the more technical questions. But Cody trusted Geoff more than she trusted doctors. She thanked him again and again.

I set up Cody's medications once a week. She took so many pills at various times during the day it was complicated to keep track of them.

During our visits Cody was not always using oxygen. She became annoyed if John, Ernie, or I confronted her about it. I did my best to convince her of its importance to her health. Occasionally I thought I got through to her. I suspected she sometimes promised to use the oxygen just to end our arguments.

Cody excitedly told Ernie about a fall auction of used Metro Mobility vans. She had lots of ideas about supplies to put in a van and colors to paint it. "We could ride with Grandma and friends in wheelchairs at the same time!"

Ernie and I attended the auction to check out the possibility. Ernie climbed under vans, opened hoods, and tested wheelchair lifts before he made a bid. To our delight, no one topped our best offer. For less than five thousand dollars Cody had a van with seats for six and spaces for three people in wheelchairs. I drove our car behind Ernie as he pulled the van into the parking lot of Cody's building. She glowed happily as he lowered the wheelchair lift so she could get inside.

Cody said owning a van made her feel like an adult. She planned as many outings in the van as she could find available drivers. One PCA especially enjoyed driving the van and spent extra hours without pay taking Cody and John to shopping malls or special events.

I purchased a finger pulse oximeter that Cody hung around her neck on a string or kept by her bed. By clipping this miniature battery-operated device on her finger, she measured her oxygen saturation in a matter of seconds. The device was expensive, but invaluable. If we argued about her use of oxygen, she used the oximeter to prove she was fine. She smiled when her saturation registered in the desirable high 90s. But when her numbers registered in the low 90s or high 80s, she'd grab for the cannula.

"Okay, okay, I'll use oxygen."

The week before Thanksgiving, Cody sent me a long email describing her complicated feelings about using oxygen:

Mom, I'm scared that I have to be on oxygen. It scares me a lot. I feel like my health is deteriorating, and that scares me. I've known that not wearing oxygen fulltime (like I should) has bothered John and makes him upset. But I didn't realize how upset until last night. He was crying into his pillow. He wouldn't let me see, or tell me why at first. He's afraid of my dying and losing me. His telling me to wear it [the cannula tubing] was getting on my nerves. But now I see why he was bugging me about it. He said things I didn't understand about my health, and I didn't know where it was coming from. Apparently he remembers everything the doctor or you have said about it. He listens to what you say, and now he is freaked out.

I've not done it 24/7 primarily because, at the time I was told I had to, I wasn't fully listening. My panic button was on. I'm still not ready, but I'm trying. The panic button goes on first, but then logic takes over (sometimes) like earlier when we talked on the phone. I understand better now, but I still don't like it. Now that I know it bothers John to the point of crying at night, and worries everyone, I will wear it all the time in the apartment. I will take it off from time to time to scratch my nose, but I won't stay off for long periods of time, unless for a good reason.

John and I both dislike doctors that generalize about me like I'm just one of those people with spina bifida, and not an individual. A thought going through my mind at the doctor's was, who is this lady? She doesn't even know me. I'm unhappy because a lot of my freedom is taken away. I don't want to go out with it yet. I don't want to be seen with it. I know I'm sick, but I don't need the whole world to know it too. Getting weird looks or being treated any differently than I already am, isn't something I'm ready to get over. You all don't notice, but I certainly do. It comes from years of knowing those looks. My own father [Dennis] gave me a look the last time he was here. I've worked hard through my life to not feel bad about being in a chair. It will take a while for me to accept the oxygen. So don't push me. I'm hoping I get used to it, like I do everything else. I think Dad is uncomfortable with my wearing oxygen—the look of it. Maybe he's just uncomfortable with me. Should I talk to Penelope about that? Or should I just write him a letter? I swear there are people who hate the look of oxygen tanks like I do. Granted, I don't want to know those people if they judge me, but I don't want to look any weaker than I already am. A woman at the doctor's office said, "Awww you poor baby" and it made me more self-conscious. I'd been sticking to my bedroom oxygen, but I'm starting today on one of the tanks. I keep reminding myself, "At least you don't need anything worse—like a respirator." This experience has made me more aware of how I react to my friend on his respirator. I talk more to him now and try to stay longer. I'm bored today—can't you tell? Sorry for the long email. I'm tired now. Talk to you later. Cody.

Cody and I talked more that evening. She sent us another email:

Hi Mom, I'm watching an exciting concert on TV. I want to see NSYNC in concert so bad, and have VIP seats. That would be awesome. I'd bring my oxygen—I don't care. I'd do anything to see them. They are so HOT. OR I'd be happy if cousin Zach came and performed the songs and danced for me. LOL. He'd probably do it to cheer me up. Hey, no teasing, ERNIE. Talk to you later. Cody

John decided to alternate holidays with his family in California. He was with Cody for Thanksgiving, so he went west for Christmas. Regrettably, this particular holiday played out the way most of 2001 had gone. Cody's shunt broke down on Christmas Eve.

Cody told each clinician, "My hair is finally long again, and I want to keep it. Shave as little as possible." The bald neurosurgeon did not empathize. Cody was devastated after surgery when she saw how much hair was gone. She whimpered, "John loved my hair."

John was terrified for Cody; his voice sounded panicked on the phone. He said he felt helpless and sorry to be so far away.

The new shunt broke down again the next day. Cody's head throbbed in pain. I lay in the dark next to her that evening while we waited for the neurosurgeon. We bemoaned that it was a heck of a way to spend Christmas night. I asked Cody if she ever became so tired of medical emergencies to the point where she thought that it would be okay to die and go to heaven. "You wouldn't have an unhealthy body in heaven. You could walk and dance."

Cody said, "No way, Mom. I don't want to die. I'm not ready for heaven yet."

I kissed her, and she asked, "Can we call Zach again?"

Zach sang on the phone for her—the same song again and again. Cody lay with her eyes shut and smiled. She said her head didn't hurt as much while Zach sang. He said a prayer that Cody's surgery would go well, and that she'd heal quickly. And that's what happened.

Two days later Cody was out of the hospital to greet John when he flew home to her.

With such a dramatic weight loss, Cody was prescribed a new wheelchair with different back support, a special seat cushion, and a new innovation in the hubs of her wheels. Ernie, now teaching night classes at a technical college, was available during the day to take Cody to appointments through the winter and spring while the chair was customized.

Cody's was still a manual chair, but the new device, activated by the push-rim of her wheel, produced a forward thrust. The extra boost made movement easier for outside wheeling. Before getting used to the feature, Cody wheeled off in unintended directions. More than once while talking on the phone, she pushed forward with one hand and I heard, "Whoaaa, hang on. I'm spinning in circles."

Wound care remained a challenge for the next year. I trained every new morning PCA and returned to do evening bandages. Two deep pressure sores were slow to heal despite my vigilance and weekly visits from a nurse. The wound care physician suggested that Cody stay in bed for three months and shift positions often throughout the day. At night, nine pillows propped her in sleep position. Even though they had a queen-size bed, there was barely room for John. The only time Cody left her bed was to see the doctor or for wheelchair fittings.

John purchased a small TV for Cody's bedroom, and Ernie bought her a laptop computer with a DVD player. He constructed a bed table for meals and craft projects. A heavy-duty cloth with pockets on the side of her bed held art supplies or personal items. When Cody wasn't watching movies or reading, she designed jewelry and cross-stitch patterns, or corresponded with Internet friends. John kept her company part of each day. Her spirits remained cheerful despite her limitations.

> Dear Mom, I'm in a slightly silly mood. How are you tonight? I wanted to tell you a few flying thoughts before I forget. 1. I couldn't get the Amy Grant tickets. :(2. Those fake bacon thingy's you bought for me are not good for me unfortunately. Too salty. At least tonight they were. 3. I have this fake mayo stuff, but no bread. What else could I put it on? It's fabulous, and I'd love to eat it. Any suggestions? 4. How's Ernie tonight? How's Blue tonight? If you want to give me a goodnight call, you may. Kiss Blue and E for me. I'll give John a kiss from all three of you. Heehee. Especially Ernie. I could just say that to see John's reaction. Naaaa. All he'll say is, "I see . . ." Thanks again for the cooking set. We finally agreed which pieces will go where. John cooked in the first piece tonight. He said it worked great. See ya. Cody

After three months in bed, Cody was allowed back in her chair. One lesion had improved but the other was worse.

Prostate cancer finally claimed Blue. Ernie and I brought him to see Cody before taking him to the vet to be put to sleep. She held her tears as she hugged the precious friend she'd found in the schoolyard almost fourteen years before. She sobbed only after we left, and John hugged her. No words could describe our grief.

For several more months I spent part of every evening helping Cody with wound care. Upon my arrival after dinner, her apartment was usually abuzz with activity—drugstore or oxygen tank deliveries, visiting friends, PCAs, and John. I stayed longer on many nights to chat with Cody after the commotion died down. I stretched out next to her on the bed. We leaned on pillows with our heads almost touching.

She told me about Internet friendships. We talked about Ernie, John, or how much we missed Blue. We joked around, remembered funny things about our dogs, and scheduled weekend activities. Cody was frustrated that she didn't have a job. Time after time health issues had interrupted her plans, interviews, and work opportunities.

One night in early May when she expressed regret about not being employed, I countered that she already had a job. "Think about it, Cody. You have a full-time job just taking care of your health. You have pills you have to remember three times a day—four times when you have bladder infections. You train and retrain PCAs on a regular basis; you track and re-order a huge inventory of medical supplies, and you schedule appointments with a half-dozen specialists. You have exercises to do, catheterization and bladder irrigation, batteries to charge, equipment to clean, and oxygen tanks to switch every few hours. On top of all that, you keep in contact with several dozen friends and relatives on the Internet and by phone. You pay bills, write letters, draw, make jewelry and cross-stitch projects, and you have John. All that doesn't even include the things you do to help your friends. I'd say you don't have time for another job."

Cody looked concerned as she said, "Laura was crying today."

Her friend Laura on the second floor was in the advanced stages of multiple sclerosis. She could maneuver her wheelchair slightly with a hand control. She'd lost her sight. She called Cody for help reaching something or taking food out of the refrigerator. When Laura had a tough day, Cody kept her company. They occasionally shared a meal.

"That's another example. The encouragement you give Laura and other friends is valuable. You're always there whenever Rachel or Gertrude needs you. You're a good listener; you give sound advice. You're a true friend who does a lot for others."

Cody said, "Christopher has been sick, and he's afraid to go to the doctor."

Christopher was an Internet friend ten years younger than Cody.

They'd corresponded for more than a year and planned to meet some-day in person. Sometimes they instant-messaged each other while watching the same TV show. According to Cody, Christopher had a tough life. He had two manual-labor-type jobs, no health insurance, and plenty of family drama. He lived in New Jersey and moved around a lot when family problems erupted. Sometimes he lived with his mother, other times with his father, sister, or grandparents. She showed me a picture of Christopher with a toddler on his lap.

"That's his nephew. He loves that kid."

"Okay then, back to my point—see what I mean? You have plenty to do without having another job."

Cody answered, "Yeah, yeah. I get it."

She signed the Mother's Day card she gave me that weekend, "It's been a fun 29 years. I love you. Cody"

Cody stopped using her BiPAP machine, saying she didn't need it any-more now that she was using oxygen 24/7. "I feel better and breathe fine without it."

Just to be safe, her cardiologist wanted Cody evaluated for sleep apnea. She had used a BiPAP for four years without actually being tested. So on a Wednesday in June, Cody's heart rate, breathing, and body movements were recorded as she slept in a sleep center that was decorated like a hotel room. Her favorite PCA spent the night with her and Cody considered the night away from home a mini-vacation with a girlfriend.

The test confirmed—Cody did not have sleep apnea. She was right about not needing a BiPAP. In fact, her health was better in general. She'd found a dependable PCA agency earlier that year and was rarely left without help. The wounds on her buttocks were almost gone and, with careful skin protection, would never return.

Chapter 28

Partners for Life

CODY'S ONLY REQUEST for her "Big Three-0" birthday party was that all her parents be there for the party at our house. I asked her what else she might want for her thirtieth birthday. So, she sent me an email with a list "in case people ask."

> $$$$$$$$$$$$$$$$$$$$$$$$$$$$$
> Harlequin romance books
> Gift cards for Target or a bookstore
> An amp with speakers
> An updated stereo with a karaoke feature
> CD changer (They are getting cheaper like Ernie said way back when.)
> Rolls of non-latex paper tape
> Rolls of quarters
> Handle tie garbage bags
> I can't think of anything else. Talk to you later. Love you. Cody

Cody and John decided to make their relationship more official. They wanted to have a commitment ceremony. She teased that they should go to Las Vegas "like Mom and Ernie did," but John said, "No. I want a wedding type of wedding."

They knew from friends that there were disadvantages to a legal marriage, reasons related to finances and disability benefits. Of their friends with disabilities who were in committed relationships, none were legally married. Legal connotations were less important to Cody and John. They wanted to say vows before God, friends, and relatives. Instead of husband and wife, they wanted to be "partners for life."

Cody wanted her family to be part of the ceremony. Her cousin Zach, now a youth pastor, accepted her request to present the vows. The date was set for the following summer on the Fourth of July 2003. Save-the-date notices went out in November inviting family and close friends to "Inter-dependence Day."

Cody called one evening to tell us about an exchange John had as they left a record store that day. She prefaced stories about her experiences with discrimination with, "Better not tell Ernie about this; you know how mad he gets when people are mean to me."

As John had followed Cody out of a store, a young guy behind the counter gestured toward John and said in a mocking tone, "There goes another one."

Recoiling at the sound of an insult, John spun his chair to face the clerk and asked in a strong voice, "Another what?"

The guy stammered, "Eh, uh, I meant another, eh, another *customer*."

Once outside the store, Cody said, "That was so good, John so brave of you to say something." John said he was proud of himself, too.

Hearing the story, Ernie's eyes flashed. "I want to get the store manager's name and complain about that guy."

Cody said, "I love Ernie. He's such a protective father."

Pals Lewis and Orlando visited Cody and John often that winter. Cody laughed, reminding them about the male stripper who came to her twenty-first birthday party. She said she was "almost" more entertained by the boys' embarrassment than by watching a sexy guy dance.

Lewis spoke with Cody alone one afternoon. There was a tender moment in their conversation when he suggested that, if Cody were not with John, Lewis would want a much closer relationship with her. Although each agreed it was too late for that, Cody described feeling both excited and slightly melancholy. She said it was "so nice to feel wanted."

As spring came, our time and attention was consumed by Inter-dependence Day preparation and visits with my mother. Mom had stopped
walking almost entirely. She and Cody sat together in their wheelchairs
in Cody's van. John folded his chair and sat in one of the seats. Now
ninety-four, Mom's memory had further faded, but her sense of humor
was intact. She joked with Cody, and every visit included singing. Mom
ended many songs with a dog-like howl. Cody urged John to howl
along, too. "*I don't know why I love you like I do, I don't know why, I just
dooooOOOOO.*"

Cody and John visited party stores to choose cake toppers, vases, and
decorations. The couple checked out reception rooms, bathrooms, and
guest rooms at a Doubletree Hotel, where an accessible room was offered
at no cost for their wedding night. The hotel chef agreed to use Ernie's
vegetarian recipe for the reception meal.

Cody and John wanted to spruce up both apartments by the time
guests came to town. John found an oak table and four chairs for his
kitchen, and drapes for his windows. Cody attacked her clutter.

Ernie offered to design a wooden wall unit in her apartment with
enough drawers and shelves for her craft supplies, books, stereo, and the
big-screen television he purchased for her the previous year. A skilled
carpenter and perfectionist, Ernie built the pieces in sections to meet
Cody's specifications. Top shelves were for decorative items and photographs. Deep drawers at the bottom were for bulky materials and files.
Small drawers were for office supplies. The oxygen concentrator fit inside
a lower section with a side opening so Cody could reach the settings and
change filters. Pickled white oak cabinetry soon covered the entire wall
on both sides of Cody's bedroom door.

Cody had a routine urology appointment in April. Dr. Lee found it
more convenient to see her at Gillette Hospital. The redecorated clinic
area now included computers for patients to use while waiting to see
the doctors. John sat with Cody as she logged onto the Internet to
scroll through photos of dogs at the Humane Society. Ever since Blue
died, Cody had tried to find a new dog for Ernie and me. She sent

emails every few days with descriptions of adorable candidates, and her plea, "I miss having a dog."

She pointed out a picture of a six-month-old puppy that looked like a young version of Blue, and looked at Ernie with hopeful eyes. A squeal escaped from Cody when he nodded and said we'd take a look at the dog after the appointment.

Cody wanted us to hurry. Ernie and I dropped off Cody and John at their apartments on the way to the Humane Society. We stopped back a short time later with our new wavy-haired puppy. Reuben ran into the apartment, jumped up on Cody, then on John. There was much hugging and licking.

Cody's friend Laura died in May. Cody and John gathered in the lobby with others from the building when they heard about it. Concerned neighbors congregated there whenever an ambulance was summoned. In a building where every tenant had a disability or medical problem, ambulances arrived all too often.

Laura's attendant of fifteen years was with her when she stopped breathing. Steve called 9-1-1 and gave her mouth-to-mouth resuscitation until paramedics arrived. He stayed in Laura's apartment as funeral plans were made. He'd be the one to clear out and distribute her things. Cody's heart went out to Steve. He had helped her over the years when she was without a PCA. She was fond of him.

> Steve, I'm concerned that you haven't been eating much. I know when you're deeply saddened, you don't feel like cooking or anything. I would like to make you something to eat tonight, tomorrow, whenever. Grilled cheese with chips? Cook up some of those things you said you have in the fridge? I'll come up and microwave them for you or cook them in the oven at John's. Whatever you want us to cook or do for you, if we can, we want to help. Talking about Laura was fun. That's how Laura would want it. I tried to call you a few minutes ago, and although I didn't get you— when trying to remember your number I was completely blank until I looked up and said, "Laura honey, if you can hear me, could you please remind me what your number was, so I could call Steve and offer to make

him something to eat?" Right then the number was right there. I think it was the number anyway, but I don't know because you didn't answer. I'm worried I may interrupt you if I come up there again—so if you need anything (talk, hug, prepared food) just call my number or John's. My parents all want to come to Laura's funeral, so please let us know when and where. On a lighter note—Please keep in touch. We want you to come to our celebration in July, so please don't disappear without letting us know where.

Hugs, Cody

Ernie and I went with Cody and John to Laura's funeral. Others from Cody's building talked in small groups and looked at table displays before the service began. Laura had been diagnosed with MS fifteen years before, soon after she finished medical school. Looking at the awards and photographs displayed on several tables, it was clear that her life until then had been full of achievement and success, world travel, and wide-ranging interests. She was accomplished in so many things that, in retrospect, it seemed she'd lived her early life faster than most people, almost as if she had to fit everything in before becoming so ill. Knowing her mostly through Cody, I saw Laura as a loving person with a strong spirit. She showed endless patience during hard times and expressed genuine kindness toward others. She reached out first to exchange a hug whenever I saw her.

Steve joined Laura's family in greeting everyone who came to the church. He was distraught, and now sick from the respiratory illness he contracted from Laura when he tried to save her. He looked weakened, tearful, and stunned. Despite the severity of Laura's illness and the progressive deterioration of her faculties, Steve said he'd always held hope that a cure for MS would be found. He loved her. In time, Steve took on some of Cody's attendant hours and she saw him almost daily.

Ernie put final touches on Cody's oak wall unit, and she put everything away just the way she wanted. She gave Ernie a cross-stitched "Happy Father's Day" with a red heart and a card.

To our father who has loved us and cared for us: We love you and cherish you. You're our hero. You're every girl and doggie's wish for a father. You make our tails and hearts flutter with great joy and happiness. We thank you for your dedication and love, and hope that you will always know how much we appreciate all you do for us. We love you. Kisses, hugs, licks, and wagging tails.

Love, Your very lucky daughter and four-legged son, Cody and Reuben

Cody collected beads and tried to interest John in beading. She showed him what to do and encouraged him to keep trying. He gave it a sporting effort despite his impaired vision, the same way he'd tried to learn how to see cross-stitch to please Cody. She eventually saw how difficult it was for him to see the tiny beads or sew little stitches. She said she loved him for trying.

Inter-dependence Day was almost upon us as Cody's daytime PCA, Kay, helped sew tiny burgundy beads onto the bodice of a full-length cream-colored dress. Cody wanted her grandmother involved in the occasion, but Mom now became agitated by noise, activity, or travel in the van. Our compromise was to put a poem of hers in the program.

There is happiness in knowing!

Do you hear the song I'm singing?
Should you catch each silent word
For me the bells are ringing!
And a song so few have heard.
The music holds such beauty
Plus a world of rainbow hues!
There's happiness in knowing
There is love and there is you!

Elma Stage Fay

Sixty-five people came to the ceremony on the Fourth of July. More than half were friends and relatives from Pennsylvania, Missouri, Georgia, North Carolina, and California.

All the children in attendance served as greeters, handing out programs and bottles of bubble soap to each guest. The program listed participants and included a "thank-you for coming" from Cody and John. Rich and Lois were listed under "John's Parents." A longer list under "Cody's Parents" included a parenthetical "Proving it takes a village . . ."

Guests took seats in rows of chairs and a few adjustments were made for friends in wheelchairs before a recording of Pachelbel's Canon began. Cody and John wheeled through doors on either side of an altar decorated with flowers and candles. Cody's eyes sparkled as she and John faced each other. He looked handsome in a blue shirt, tie, and slacks. Cody glowed in her long dress and matching shoes. Burgundy flower buds on her headband matched the tiny beads on her bodice.

Charlie stood and offered a welcome. He described the couple's "tender-hearted" relationship. "This is a story of a long distance Internet romance that grew to become a blending of two hearts into a strong, sincere love. Those of you who know them well know that in many ways these two people are miracles of God. He gave them life. He sustained them during some tough times. And now, He has given them to each other."

Cody and John smiled. Charlie said a prayer asking God to bless the partnership. Lewis's mother, Cynthia, sang "When You Say Nothing At All." She learned Cody and John's "song" just for the occasion. As candles were lit, Julie read about love from I Corinthians.

When Zach stood to speak, he said how much he cared about Cody and John, that they were "an example of true love. They fell in love so many years ago and committed to each other even before they met in person." He shared entertaining anecdotes about the couple and wove their love story into a larger message about the love Jesus has for each of us.

Zach asked, "Cody and John, do you promise to love each other unfailingly, support and respect each other faithfully, and serve God and each other as long as you live?" Both said yes and wheeled forward so their chairs were parallel as they helped each other put on matching gold rings. With arms in an embrace, they kissed. Guests clapped and cheered.

After Zach and Julie sang a duet, Charlie concluded, "Tonight, you will see fireworks celebrating the birth of our great nation, fireworks that will sparkle and brighten up the night. Tonight, and in the years ahead whenever you see fireworks, no matter what the occasion, think of Cody and John and send a prayer their way. Pray that the sparkle of love that you see in their eyes right now will become contagious to those around them and continue forever."

As Charlie presented the "partners for life," Ernie began to play the piano. Sheets with lyrics were included in the programs and everyone sang "Could I Have This Dance." The ceremony ended with hundreds of rainbow bubbles floating down around Cody and John.

Guests greeted the couple, nibbled hors d'oeuvres and sipped drinks before gathering in the adjoining reception room. A deejay played soft music during dinner. Conversation and laughter filled the room. Ernie offered the first toast and, on behalf of Cody and John, thanked everyone for coming. Tad stood and described his annual summer visits to the State Fair with the couple. He called John "Pathfinder" and toasted him as a good choice as Cody's partner for life. Gertrude stood and said that Cody was her best friend, and now John was also her best friend.

John's closest friends since grade school sat together. They had gone out for drinks the night before with John. Cody had joined them later in the evening.

One man stood and said, "I want to speak on behalf of John's California friends." He said their friendship had spanned many years and, as each of them had finished school and gone on to jobs and marriage, the friends often wondered what would happen to John. They hoped for him to have similar good fortune. And now, having met Cody, they were pleased that John would also know the same happiness.

Cake and festive music followed, and expressive dancing that was not confined to couples or fancy footwork. With a half-dozen people in wheelchairs, there were all kinds of movements. A few people who started the evening with inhibitions appeared to lose them in the rhythm and excitement. Whenever an Abba song played, Charlie's wife Edie waved her scarf and danced in turn with everyone on the dance floor. Dennis held Cody's hands and spun her around and under his arms. Cody's face was flushed with happiness. She and John danced, hugged, and kissed.

As the sun began to set, guests took their drinks outdoors to watch ground-level fireworks in the hotel parking lot. Tad brought a guitar outside and people sang folksongs. Cody and John held sparklers and watched twirling firecrackers. When it was almost fully dark, rumbles were heard in the distance. Guests took elevators to the high floors of the hotel where full-length windows made it possible to view firework displays in every direction from downtown Minneapolis and five suburbs.

The evening ended with warm goodbyes and reminders to out-of-town guests to come to the lunch at our house the following day. Ernie and I loaded the car with flowers and gifts.

Before leaving for the night we went to Cody and John's hotel room. Tad and his brother Ty had also stopped by to say goodnight. Cody was tired but still beaming as she and John sat together on the bed. Cody's attendant, Kay, had the room next door so she'd be available to help Cody in the morning.

Sometime before midnight Cody and John were hungry and called room service to order food. But the kitchen staff had been allowed to go home early due to the holiday, so Kay offered to take them to a restaurant. While positioning Cody's wheelchair to strap it in the van, a dangling seat belt caught on something and flew up. The metal end smacked Cody in the head and she cried out in pain. She spent the rest of the night cradled in John's arms. He stayed awake worrying that the blow might have affected her shunt. But all was well by morning. Cody told me that the way John held her through the night was the sweetest feeling she ever had.

Cody and John radiated wistful contentment in the days that followed. Inter-dependence Day had been a success and they enjoyed recalling the details. They laughed about the funny parts, reveled in the wonderful things family and friends had said to them, and appreciated that so many traveled so far to be with them.

Chapter 29

Side Effects

JOHN AND CODY spent some wedding gift cash on DVDs. I offered Cody a dollar per DVD to borrow a few. Some weeks later I received this email:

Subject: DVD Rental Late Fees

Dear Ms. Cornell

This is to inform you of the late fee for the 6 DVDs you rented from Cody's Rental in Downtown Hopkins. Since it has been three weeks since your first rental, the dollar-a-DVD for a week is now 3 dollars a DVD if not paid in full by the end of the day today. Thank you for choosing Cody's Rental for your finest DVD watching. I look forward to serving you again soon.

Sincerely, Cody J. Ahlburg (Founder & Co-founder & Owner)

P.S. We love you

More and more, Cody found it necessary to plan her day around the side effects of Lasix. The strong diuretic made her pee every twenty minutes for at least two hours each time she took it. Taking such a high dose twice a day made staying dry a challenge. Dr. Lee suggested a medicated patch to increase Cody's bladder capacity, but she didn't want to risk more side effects.

When the four of us went to see *Mama Mia* in December, she took Lasix early in the day. Even so, she had to leave the performance twice to go to the restroom. However, Cody rocked to the Abba songs and enjoyed the musical about a girl with three possible fathers, one being Australian. She quipped, "That was like the story of my life!"

Because Lasix leeched potassium from her body, Cody took a

potassium supplement. When a blood test in January revealed an iron deficiency, she started taking a supplement for that as well. Both iron and potassium caused constipation and discomfort. Her doctor suggested eating red meat for more iron.

Cody told him, "Eating animals doesn't make me feel good."

But she was finally so uncomfortable that she agreed to eat meat. John prepared beef liver for her, but they both said it was "gross." Ernie and I brought her frozen steaks and free-range meat. However, Cody's iron tested too low no matter how much meat she consumed in the coming months.

That spring Cody told me, "John's really nervous about something. You should talk to him. He thinks that you and Ernie will send him back to California if I die."

Startled, I asked, "What? What's that about? Why would he think that?"

She urged, "Call him. He's in his apartment."

I called John and asked him to explain. He said Cody told him that she'd die if she needed another shunt surgery. He worried that Ernie and I would no longer help him if Cody died, and he'd have to return to California.

I addressed one point at a time. "First, Cody *will* probably have more shunt surgeries. But there's no reason to think that another shunt operation would be fatal. Second, you're an adult; you decide for yourself where you live. Third, if Cody died, Ernie and I would help you do what *you* want to do. If you want to go back to California, we'd help you do that. If you want to stay in Minnesota, we'd help you to do that. It's all up to you."

After a pause, John said, "Okay. That's good. I was worried. I don't want to go back there to live. Getting around here is easier; transportation and other services for the handicapped are better."

"Ernie and I aren't going anywhere, John. But even if we both died tomorrow, there's nothing we do for you that you couldn't figure out how to do. You have friends, and there are county social workers and agencies that provide services for blind people. There are all kinds of ways to get help. You already know about those things, right?"

"Yeah, I guess so. I was just worried."

Now I needed to call back Cody.

She explained to me, "I thought after that last surgery that you said I'd die if I had to have another shunt revision."

Horrified, I tried to think of what I'd said that could have given her such an impression. The closest thing I could remember was explaining to Cody that if her shunt broke down at the lower end, where tubing went into a vein, it was a more complicated surgery than replacing the top part that went into her head. I explained it again and clarified that this didn't mean it was fatal.

"My gosh, Cody. Have you been worried about this for a long time?"

"Well, yeah."

"Cody, you need to tell me when you worry about stuff like that."

The next day Cody reported that John was relieved to hear that Ernie and I would still be around for him if she died. She chuckled. "I think he was more relieved about that than he was to find out I won't die if I need another shunt surgery."

In April Cody moved into a freshly painted apartment across the hall. After living in the front of the building for a decade, she was ready for a quieter environment. Outside were trees instead of a noisy parking lot. She could open windows without smelling diesel exhaust from Metro Mobility buses. The floor plan was identical to her original apartment, but we all had to get used to turning left instead of right in the hallway. Cody was pleased. "I like this place. It's clean."

The week of her move, a routine urology exam and ultrasound confirmed diminished bladder capacity and a small kidney stone. Dr. Lee didn't think the stone was a problem for the moment, but he talked with Cody about her difficulties staying dry. In order to sleep through the night, she now paper-taped her catheter in the Mitrofanoff opening, like an indwelling catheter, attached to a drainage bag by the bed. Still, she often leaked onto the bedding. John awoke at some point almost every night to help her change clothes. If he had to change sheets, he was up for at least an hour. They were both cranky from sleep deprivation. Dr. Lee again recommended the medicated patch to expand her bladder capacity.

Cody insisted, "I'm afraid of that medicine. I read that a side effect is constipation, and that's already a bad problem for me. Plus, I don't want to feel groggy."

Dr. Lee acknowledged that side effects were possible but he wanted her to try it anyway. If the patch didn't help, another bladder augmentation surgery was a possibility. When Cody heard "surgery," she agreed to try the patch.

Cody took many medications, all of which had side effects. Some were minor, but a side effect of one medication caused a near-fatal incident when her shunt broke down that summer.

Because Cody was taking a blood-thinning drug, immediate brain surgery couldn't be done without risk of a hemorrhage. The neurosurgeon delayed operating until another medication could counteract the blood thinner. Hours passed as Cody's head pain increased. I stayed with her in the ER, and many more hours in the ICU. In misery, she opened her eyes only to tell each resident to make sure that no one cut away much of her hair, now long past her shoulders.

Seeing suddenly that Cody faded out of consciousness, a resident grabbed a resuscitator bag. The doctors couldn't wait any longer. Someone squeezed the blue airbag every few seconds as clinicians rushed alongside Cody's gurney to the O.R. All I could do was pray and hold my fear.

Hours later Cody was brought back to the ICU. The anesthesiologist had trouble waking her after surgery, so she remained on a respirator. There was no room for a cot or wheelchair in the ICU, so John stayed home. Ernie arrived to trade places with me. But I wanted to stay while Cody was on the respirator. Her eyes pleaded as she gestured to have the ventilator tubing removed from her throat. She was conscious and uncomfortable for several hours. The resident in charge said Cody was retaining too much carbon dioxide to consider taking it out. He agreed finally to do another blood test in a couple of hours to see if her CO_2 level normalized.

Ernie assured the doctor that we supported Cody's request to have the respirator removed as he described Cody's hypoventilation. But the resident insisted that the CO_2 level in her blood was dangerously high; he didn't want to risk it. I asked who else we could speak to with the authority to remove it. He called in the chief resident, who was just as resolute. He tried to impress upon Cody, and us, the serious consequences of removing the respirator if she still couldn't breathe on her own. I repeated that Cody's CO_2 was much higher than normal at best and, if he insisted on waiting for it to be "normal," she could be on a respirator *for the rest of her life.*

Cody used a pen and wrote, "I want this out. Now! Take it out. I'll be fine. Take it out."

The doctor agreed to a blood test right away, promising that if he saw any change, he'd remove the machine. The test showed only slight improvement, but we held him to his word. He said this was against his better judgment and we shouldn't be surprised if he had to put Cody right back on a respirator. But once the tubing was removed, Cody was comfortable and breathed normally. The astonished doctor said, "If you or I had that level of CO_2 in our blood, we'd be dead."

I thought of the tigers that lived for many years at the Bronx Zoo, breathing exhaust from cars and trucks on nearby highways. The lead level in the animals' blood was so high that scientists said the tigers should have been dead. After so many years, the tigers had adapted to lethal amounts of poison.

Knowing she could need emergency brain surgery again at some point, Cody didn't feel safe taking blood-thinning medication ever again. In light of the close call, none of her doctors objected to her decision.

Two test results during Cody's hospitalization were heartening. No pulmonary hypertension was detected and her echocardiogram was normal. On the other hand, the entire left side of her head was shaved front to back. Cody's request had been ignored. She was more than despondent. She told me to cut off the rest of her long hair and she began to cry.

"It'll grow back, sweetie. You've always looked cute with short hair. The bald look is kind of in style. Lots of people shave their heads on purpose."

Cody was serious and angry as she said, "I will never grow my hair long again."

Tears stung my eyes as I saw how dispirited she was to lose her beautiful long hair. I cut away the rest and saved a lock for John.

Two weeks later, Cody had another bad headache. She took migraine medicine and the pain subsided. The headache came and went for another two weeks. Just as we'd think it must be her shunt, the pain disappeared for a day or so. Cody saw her primary care doctor twice, but the headache cycle persisted. Stress was building between Cody and John. He worried constantly, and worry made him irritable. He checked on her continually, asking about her headache again and again. Cody said his worry was driving her crazy. Fears overlapped and erupted into arguments. She sent John to his apartment during the day or he'd leave on his own. Each reached out to Internet friends for relief from tension that escalated along with the headache pain.

One evening I found a couple of unopened bills on Cody's kitchen counter and more in her oxygen tank bag. This was unusual. Cody had always paid her bills in a timely manner. She was embarrassed and cranky to see evidence of poor recordkeeping. Now, my fear was building.

Every morning that summer, I arrived at work to see the message light blinking on my phone. Each time, my heart jumped. There was always at least one call from Cody. She left messages in the middle of the night and early in the morning. I ached as I listened to her tales of misery and difficulty or heard her cry into the phone. I called her back and we decided what to do about whatever the trouble was that day. Problems ranged from painful constipation, blood in her urine, low-grade fevers, nausea, allergic reactions, and so on. Some problems required calls or visits to doctors. On a day when her head hurt again, I set up an appointment with her neurosurgeon. Cody's cousin Joanna, now sixteen, was visiting from Missouri later that week and Cody had plans for fun.

The neurosurgeon didn't examine Cody and seemed unconcerned. He didn't think her headaches were shunt-related. As he spoke, Ernie and I exchanged glances. We told him how miserable Cody had been and continued to press for advice. Finally, at our request, he ordered a CAT scan. The test showed slightly enlarged ventricles, but the doctor didn't think surgery was warranted; the symptoms might be from a migraine. He sent her home.

Joanna stayed with Ernie and me during her visit and spent her days with Cody and John. They went out to eat, worked on craft projects together, and talked for hours. One evening when I came to pick up Joanna, Cody called me into her bedroom. She burst into tears, saying she hated feeling so awful while her cousin was there. I hugged her and told her how sorry I was that she felt miserable. I wanted so badly to cheer her up. I suggested, "Maybe you can try to think of it this way: Even though you feel crummy, you're with your sweet cousin. Doesn't having Joanna here make you feel a little better than you would otherwise?" Cody said that was true.

Two days after Joanna's visit, Cody's eyes were sunsetting; she was completely unable to look up. I called 9-1-1. Before paramedics arrived, Cody phoned my brother Charlie for a prayer and to ask Zach to call her at the hospital.

By now we had the same system for emergencies. John stayed home until there was concrete information about Cody's condition. He preferred not to spend the first night; with his vision impairment he was afraid he might miss something important while she was so vulnerable. That was fine with me. I wanted to be with Cody during the scariest parts of emergencies to make sure information was shared with the right people and to know she was safe. Once she was stable I could sleep. John was loving and attentive company for Cody once the emergency part was done.

Ernie went home to sleep while Cody and I readied for the night in the ER cubicle. When Zach called, Cody held the phone to her ear for more than an hour as he said prayers and sang to her. She kept her eyes shut and smiled even while her head hurt. They were giggling by the time she hung up.

Hours later, Cody began to cry. "I have been so mean to John lately, and I'm so sorry. I want to call and tell him."

"Cody, it's 2:30 in the morning. John's probably asleep."

She sobbed, "I have to tell him I love him."

I dialed John's number and Cody cried to John that she was sorry for being so crabby lately. She promised, "You're the one I love. If I die, you can have my big-screen TV."

She talked to John for twenty minutes, professing love and her regrets for misdeeds. He said similar loving things to her.

When Cody hung up I said, "You're funny, telling John he could have your TV if you die. You told Ernie the same thing before he went home."

Cody laughed and said, "Oops!"

Before dawn Cody was groggy and melancholy again. She opened her eyes for a moment and said, "I love you, Mom. If I die in surgery . . ."

I was the third person she said could have her big-screen TV.

The sun was up by the time Cody was wheeled to the pre-op area. The neurosurgeon on call was a new addition to the medical staff. He'd come from Philadelphia. Cody smiled hearing the doctor was from her hometown. He was a heavyset middle-aged fellow with a flushed complexion. He spoke in warm tones, assuring Cody that he'd done this surgery many times. He promised to take good care of her.

Cody said, "I feel better just knowing you're from Philly." But when he left she whispered, "He doesn't look healthy. I hope he doesn't collapse during my surgery."

By noon Cody was on the phone to John, family, and friends to say the operation went well. John spent the night with Cody and she was home the next day.

Cody and John were feeling close and happy again. She took a renewed interest in her exercise schedule, craft projects, and a stringed instrument she bought the previous year at the State Fair.

Two weeks later *another* headache came and went intermittently. Discouraged, Cody asked the doctor from Philly to be her new neurosurgeon. She did not want to ever again see the doctor who shaved her head. In one week she'd turn thirty-two; Cody didn't want a shunt problem to ruin her plans for a birthday visit from her uncle and aunt. Charlie and Edie were coming to take Cody and John to a Gloria Estefan concert.

The Philly doctor said he appreciated her request but admitted he was baffled by her recurring headaches. He wanted her to see his senior associate, the head of the neurosurgery department, Dr. Haines. We felt new hope that there might be a wiser expert who could help end this painful cycle. The earliest available appointment with Dr. Haines was a few weeks later in September.

Chapter 30

Fear and Faith

THE DAY BEFORE her birthday, Cody sent a group email to John, some friends, and me: "I'm not superstitious, but this is very true and sweet, plus I could use some good luck. Talk to all of you soon who I send this to. Love you."

The attached story was about a man whose wife had just died. He found some unused clothing she'd saved many years for a "special occasion." The message said not to put off good things for a day that may never come; live each day as though it were already a special occasion.

Cody whimpered that her head hurt as she wheeled from her van to attend the Gloria Estefan performance at the Target Center. I leaned down and said a quick prayer that she'd be able to enjoy her birthday concert. My fears were rising along with further distress that Cody was in pain and, again, I couldn't fix it.

Cody's friend Sharon joined Cody and John in the handicapped section. They rocked together with the music. Sharon held her hand over Cody's eyes to protect her from the bright strobe lights. When the concert ended, Sharon joined the rest of us in the van. Even though Cody's head hurt, she smiled and laughed as we drove Sharon home.

Birthday "season" continued with visits from more out-of-town relatives. Near the end of a visit from John's parents, Cody described a pain near her clavicle. The area was hot, red, and swollen around a small scar near the shunt tubing.

As usual, Cody and I spent all night in the ER and the "Philly" neuro-surgeon performed a shunt revision the next morning. But Cody was re-admitted three days later when swelling and redness on her neck worsened. Cody sat in her wheelchair next to the bed in a small hospital room as we waited to meet with the senior neurosurgeon, Dr. Haines.

The tall man with gray at the temples walked into the room, intro-duced himself, and sat down in a chair facing Cody. He adjusted his glasses and read the medical summary I handed him. He looked directly at Cody as he asked her questions, and appeared relaxed as he listened to her description of what had gone on over the summer and her worries about the recurring headaches. The doctor's calm demeanor and respect-ful attention inspired confidence.

Dr. Haines remained thoughtful for a moment before recommending a course of action. He suspected that Cody had a long-term low-grade infection, which had probably not been detected before now because the offending bacteria took awhile to show up in a blood culture. Dr. Haines wanted to test her blood further and remove Cody's shunts—both shunts. The one on the right side of her head had not functioned since she was fifteen. His premise was that bacteria had attached to the plastic shunt apparatus. All plastic had to come out for at least a week. In the meantime, Cody would have an externalized shunt, a sterile tube drain-ing cerebrospinal fluid from her head. Her blood would be tested daily while she was given aggressive IV antibiotics. Once bacteria no longer appeared in blood cultures, she'd get a new shunt.

As we listened to Dr. Haines I felt a surge of hope. He'd given Cody's case genuine thought and consideration. What he said made sense. How-ever, Cody's face showed increased panic as she realized that Dr. Haines was suggesting two surgeries, and she'd be confined to a small space in a hospital room, attached to tubing. She burst into tears. I moved to her side and tried to reassure her, but she was distraught.

She cried, "I'm scared. I'm afraid I'll die."

Dr Haines leaned forward with his elbows on his knees and said in a matter-of-fact voice, "Oh, this won't kill you. This will just be very bor-ing for you. You will be bored and frustrated, but then you'll be better."

He stayed to answer her questions and reassure her about the course of treatment. By the time he left, Cody was resigned to the plan. She wasn't happy, but she understood the intent and the promise of a positive outcome. The best news for Cody was that Dr. Haines did not support the notion that brain surgery required hair removal. He cited studies that demonstrated that this standard precaution had not been proven to make a difference in the incidents of postoperative infections. *If only we'd found this doctor years sooner!*

Ernie arrived later in the evening with a laptop, books, and art supplies for Cody. She had concerns to ask Dr. Haines about the following morning before surgery. Ernie wrote them on the back of a hospital menu.

- I'm very sensitive. I'm afraid of being left alone; I panic.
- I'm afraid they'll be mean to me in post-op. Please get me off the respirator right away ASAP after surgery. I hypoventilate (retain CO_2 & have abnormal blood gases)
- Have you ever run into this same situation before?
- [Ernie added] How is the tube that replaces the shunt not going to be contaminated?

I slept that night on a cot next to Cody's bed. She reached for my hand. She squeezed my fingers every once in a while as we each drifted in and out of sleep. Sometime in the middle of the night we were both awake in the dark. For the moment, there was no fear. Cody spoke in a wistful singsong voice. "You know, Mom. I was thinking about Dr. Haines and his idea for two surgeries. I thought—*two surgeries . . . hmmm . . . That would mean two invoices for Dr. Haines.*" She paused briefly, then said, "I see Jamaica . . . I see Hawaii . . ."

Dr. Haines provided informative answers to the questions the next morning and encouraged Cody not to worry. Just as he predicted, the removal of the shunts was quick. Cody was back in her room with a transparent tube extending from her head to a clear plastic bag that hung at a measured distance from an IV pole. A PICC line was put under her right arm for frequent blood draws. She wasn't allowed to change position without adjusting the level of the drainage bag to ensure that her intracranial pressure remained constant. Ernie and I learned how to make the adjustment.

Early the following morning, Cody and John were frightened when a lab tech who came to take blood tried to insert a needle in the sterile tube coming from Cody's head. Cody argued and struggled with the woman for a few minutes until a nurse entered the room and shouted for the lab tech to "STOP!"

Other than the mishap with the lab tech, and the associated incident report, the next week was uneventful. John, Ernie, and I alternated spending nights with Cody. Dennis visited. Steve and other friends came by, but Cody's room was too small for another wheelchair. John had to maneuver around the room on crutches.

I took the hospital shuttle from my office to visit Cody or spend the night with her. She thanked Ernie and me each day for every effort we made to ease her boredom and discomfort. She said she wished we didn't have to do so much for her. We wondered together about these last few months of surgeries and headache pain, and tried to think of some larger life lesson we were supposed to be learning from the unremitting stress and strain. I suggested, "Maybe this happened to help you see how much you're loved by John and your parents." She said she'd thought about that, too.

Each time I entered her room, Cody told me whether her nurse on that shift was wonderful (warm, friendly and helpful), so-so (impersonal, just doing a joyless job) or horrible (crabby, disrespectful, sloppy, or rough). If a nurse was in the room when I arrived, Cody signaled with her facial expression which type it was. A good nurse made a huge difference in every aspect of each day in the hospital.

On the last day of September the blood cultures were clear; the infection was gone. Dr. Haines operated. For the first time since age fifteen, Cody had VP shunt tubing that extended to her abdominal region instead of to her heart. Dennis, Ernie, and I greeted her together when she came out of recovery.

Cody smiled. She said she felt "terrific. I can think straight again."

She had to remain on IV vancomycin for another week. She could go home if she had a family member who could administer IV dosages.

That wasn't me—not my level of comfort or expertise. I knew how frequently IVs became obstructed and how the area around needles could become sore. Dennis was not a candidate either in light of his tendency to faint around needles. The only one who could have done it was Ernie. But he had developed a virulent chest cold on the last day of Cody's hospital stay. He didn't want to risk her health by being near her while he was so sick.

The alternative was a seven-day stay in the transitional care unit, a cross between a hospital and a hotel, located in a building near my office. John and I alternated nights with Cody. I came to see her before work, joined her for lunch, and returned at the end of my workday. She was itching to get out and about. Sometimes I brought her to my office or took her for a walk around the hospital campus. But then I caught whatever Ernie had.

John spent the last few nights with Cody before her discharge. Ernie and I were the walking wounded when we drove her home to her apartment.

I couldn't join Cody for her follow-up appointment with Dr. Haines; I was sick in bed. My head was exploding; I had nonstop coughing fits, a daily fever, neck pain, and endless congestion. I briefly considered that God had chosen for me to die of this illness. I was not feeling so confident anymore that God's life purpose for me was caring for Cody. I lay in bed thinking about the pain I felt during the proceeding four months—the stress and fear, seeing my daughter suffer. The hardest part of it was when her spirit wavered, when she felt depressed under the weight of her troubles. That was a rarity for Cody. She was brave and strong; it took a lot to discourage her. I wondered why I became so sick just as she was able to come home from the hospital. She needed me for various things, but I couldn't help. I could barely eek out a whisper to speak.

As we prepared questions by phone for her appointment with Dr. Haines, I whispered to Cody, "Maybe this sickness is God's way of insisting that I let go of my ongoing attempts to fix all things Cody."

"I had that same thought, Mom. It's okay. I'm fine seeing Dr. Haines alone."

I emailed my brother Charlie:

> I have not seen Mom in a month. I feel terrible about it. I called there each
> week, until I lost my voice, to make sure she's fine, but I know she misses the
> music and hugs. I doubt I can visit her until the weekend after this one to be
> safe. Even Ernie isn't really well yet—he still coughs at night too and tires eas-
> ily. It was weird to be with Cody day after day, and sleep with her every third
> night, then every other night when Ernie got so sick. Then I was cut off! Not
> seeing her at all in a week feels so weird. We sure had some sweet chats in
> the middle of the night. She went through such a difficult series of proce-
> dures, tests, and daily discomforts—as usual impressing me with her basic
> spirit. I am amazed she stayed healthy. It's so hard to get any sleep in the hos-
> pital—they came in ALL THE TIME for neuro checks, blood, and all manner of
> interruption. I obviously am paying the price for the missed rest!

Cody took good care of herself during our time apart. She called Tad, her
grandmother, aunts, uncles, cousins, and friends. Her fingers flew across
her keyboard as she contacted Internet pals and reported her good health.
I was well enough to visit her the next week. We spent an evening making jewelry. We strung beads and assembled necklaces. Cody taught me
how to attach wires and clasps. We spent another evening separating a
two-gallon container of plastic beads by color. The project was satisfying
for Cody and surprisingly satisfying for me, too.

Cody was concerned about something she felt in her abdomen. Feeling
the area, I wondered if it was scar tissue from the operation. She tried
unsuccessfully to reach Dr. Haines by phone, so she sent him an email.

> I am experiencing firmness in the area directly under the incision in my
> stomach where you put the bottom of my VP shunt on September 30th.
> I first noticed it a few days ago, and to me it feels a little firmer. My fear is
> that spinal fluid is collecting there. I am having a CAT scan of my abdomen
> tomorrow for my urologist at Gillette. I will ask him if he sees anything out
> of the ordinary. He also works at the U. It would make me feel much better
> to know what your opinion is of this so please email me with your advice

or call me. I am fine in all other ways. I do not have a headache, or any other of my shunt malfunction symptoms. I look forward to hearing from you. Thank you for your time. Cody J. Ahlburg

P.S. In case you have trouble remembering me, I am the spina bifida patient, who had the blood infection, and always had lots of questions for you. You were right. I didn't die and it was very long, and boring, and frustrating just like you said.

Dr. Haines emailed back that evening, "Cody—I have no trouble remembering you." He explained that many people experience a firm lump at this point after a shunt is replaced. He said it was probably not a problem, but he thought it would be useful for him to see the CAT scan.

In the spirit of Cody's new decision to handle medical appointments on her own, she asked Steve to drive John and her to the urology appointment in St. Paul. Steve had been Cody's evening PCA frequently and sometimes her daytime PCA since Laura died.

Cody had a list of questions for Dr. Lee. She was particularly concerned that he might recommend another bladder surgery to address the continuing leakage. She said she'd been irrigating her bladder daily and using the patch for three months with little improvement.

After the CAT scan, Dr. Lee explained the results. There was fluid under her abdomen incision; another pocket of fluid "of unknown source" was found in her pelvic region; a large stone needed to be removed from her right kidney. She had smaller stones in both kidneys and a large number of stones in the bladder.

Cody panicked. John panicked. Steve held her hand. She called me at work on her cell phone.

Her voice shook as she said, "Mom. This is not looking good."

My stomach began to flip the way it always had when there was a new reason for fear. After all the events of the past five months, these new developments seemed too huge. I decided in that instant that none of us could respond with fear anymore. God had a plan and, whatever this was, it would get worked out somehow.

"Cody, we need to stop letting fear get the best of us. I am going to repeat to myself to trust God on this, and I want you to do the same."

Her voice calmed down as she said, "Okay."

Feeling like a warrior discussing combat strategy, I told Cody, "This fear we keep having with every emergency is huge. It must be stopped. Let's take this one step at a time and find out what we need to do. Can I talk to Dr. Lee?"

Dr. Lee explained the problems and potential solutions. Cody needed two surgeries—first to remove bladder stones, and a few weeks later to remove the large kidney stone. Surgery was necessary. The kidney stone could be taken out with a scope through a tiny insertion from the back. He said we'd talk more in a few days.

Cody and I spoke again that evening and vowed together to try to stay calm. I said, "God has a plan. We have to resist the temptation to be scared about this."

While praying in times of stress, I often found an important message by choosing a random verse from the Bible. My finger landed that night on Psalm 28:6–7. As I read the verse I felt waves of angel shivers on my arms and back.

Oh, praise the Lord, for he has listened to my pleadings! He is my strength, my shield from every danger. I trusted in him, and he helped me. Joy rises in my heart until I burst out in songs of praise to him. (The Living Bible)

Thank you, God. Please help Cody and me to keep faith.

Cody went with a PCA to deliver the CAT scan to Dr. Haines. I offered to find out when the bladder stone removal could be scheduled. Cody focused on more interesting things for a few days. One of her PCAs hosted a "passion" party and Cody purchased several items to spark up her love life with John. She called and emailed Tad and her friends, shopped at bead stores, and tried not to think about operations.

The first available date for bladder surgery was two weeks later on the first Friday in November. Cody thought that was too soon, but agreed to it when I pointed out two advantages. First, she wouldn't have much time to worry if it was over with soon; and second, she could have both surgeries out of the way before the holidays.

Nine days before the scheduled surgery, she sent this email:

Subject: I need understanding:

Mom, I'm still confused. Why do I need more major surgery? What are they going to do to me, and why? I just don't want to go through anything that is life threatening. Is this the type of thing you get a second opinion? Do you still feel good about everything? Yeah, I don't like surgery, but whatever is going on has to be fixed, and I just want the easiest thing done. Please explain in an email what's going on with me. TY

I wrote a long email describing each concern in detail. I explained the alternatives we'd been told about and the planned procedures. She'd be in the hospital for three days. I stressed that an important aspect of the bladder surgery was to find out what the fluid was near the shunt incision. Dr. Lee called the operation "open cystolithotomy and drainage of peritoneal fluid." He considered it a "maintenance" procedure. I urged Cody to have faith in Dr. Lee and God that she'd be fine, that it's another annoying thing, but the result will be good. I ended with, "Let me know if this summary helps you understand it better. I love you. Mom."

Yeah, it helped me unerstand. I was impressed that John asked Dr. Lee some questions. Love you, Cody

P.S. Dad [Dennis] emailed and said I should write a book about how to be a good patient in the hospital, or something like that.

Cody called that night asking again why surgery had to be done right away. I reminded her that it wasn't an emergency; she could decide for herself when to have the operation. I didn't see her other email until the next morning.

Mom, Why is it such a rush now, when in the office Dr. Lee acted as if it was no big deal? Why do I have to do it so soon? Don't get me wrong, hey, get the things out of there, but what happened to letting me heal from the head one, and letting me have some fun before giving me a scare? I'm not comfortable with that. Did something change, and I'm not getting it yet? John is unhappy with the doctor for making me do it right away. Yeah, John isn't a calm person, and neither am I, but Lee said, "Okay we'll do this sometime in a few months." We all said "Hey cool, thanks"

I was scared and hung onto Steve, but was okay with the understanding of a few months. The part I don't get is, why the rush? You probably said it already. I'll read it again, cause who knows.

I emailed back:

Hi Cody, As I said last night, it's not a huge rush. Before it was scheduled, we both agreed it would be good to get it over with. Plus, yesterday morning you said you were miserable from the bloating. If you're feeling bad from any of this—I think the sooner the better to get it fixed. You'll have it over with and enjoy the holidays without this stuff to worry about. If Dr. Lee is correct, your bladder will work better and have more capacity, so your overall quality of life will improve.

As of Monday, November 1, Cody still planned to go through with surgery on Friday.

Chapter 31

One Week

TUESDAY

AT THE PRE-OP APPOINTMENT Cody asked her primary care doctor how urgent it was for her to have the bladder stones removed. The doctor didn't think it mattered too much and affirmed that it was her choice. The majority of Cody's forty-plus hospitalizations and surgeries were on an emergency basis. She was not used to having a choice.

Cody thought the preparation for surgery was repulsive. She had to drink a chalky mixture and have an enema the night before. She grappled with the decision to postpone the operation. She emailed her friend Sharon, saying that she wasn't sure she'd make it through the surgery. She emailed Dennis that night.

> Hi Dad, How long will you be in town? You're in town now right? I am really scared about Friday. I have to go through a lot of unbelievably bad stuff before it. It's stuff I can't even stomach. Do you have any time to spend with me Wed night? I realize my request is kind of short notice, but I'm really stressed. I know you're not sure about my health anymore, but I'm not as strong as I used to be. I'm not able to do a lot I used to. It's scary to me, cause I like to do things myself. I'd like you to come over—maybe meet you for lunch or something. Let me know what you are doing, and if you're available. Hey, did you ever contact your wife about what she wrote to me? Someone I know explained to me what the phrase was supposed to mean. It's still funny to me. Ah, that Penelope, she's so funny. Even when she wasn't planning to be, I don't think? Talk soon. Love you, CJ

Cody emailed me a half hour later:

> Mom, You've always said I couldn't have enemas. When we said it tonight,
> we didn't stop to think, uh, my ass will fall out, or something bad will
> happen. I'm just not comfortable with how things are coming along. I
> need more time to think. This was pushed against me, and too much has
> to be okay with me before time will run out. I want to be healthy, but also
> mentally safe and happy. That is hard right now. Please help me undo it
> for this week. I know you probably have it all set up with work and stuff,
> but all this is moving too fast. I need kidneys, but they have been in
> trouble for a while, and they aren't even what's being taken care of first.
> Oh, and today I would have liked a CAT scan to see if anything changed.
> I didn't speak up because [PCA] was waiting in the van. She was po'd as
> it was late when we got out there I think. Anyway, this is how I feel. Don't
> think lightly here. Cody

I called Cody again to assure her it was her decision, that I would truly not
be inconvenienced either way and she was free to make up her own mind.

WEDNESDAY

> Daddy, I'm scared. I need to do a lot that I had to do with the first bladder
> surgery. I'll tell you all about it tonight. Well, there will probably be three
> of us. Um, I have Steve with me 5–7 p.m., and he's been really sweet and
> supportive through a lot of things with me lately, so it's your decision.
> With him and John, it could be four if you don't care—although John
> and I have been through a tough time the last couple days. Let me know
> what you want to do. I'm highly upset, so be nice to me please (not that
> you aren't always) No stress aloud [sic]. I love you.

A few minutes later she emailed John's brother's family:

> Hi everyone. Yeah, I'm ok. Scared out of my mind, but hey, maybe I'll
> be comforted by having a nurse that looks like Jennifer again. I wish I
> remembered the woman's name. Oh well. Anyway, I saw John's email
> cause he showed me, so I thought I'd respond on my own. I go in early
> Friday morning. They say I'll be home by Sunday, but my response is, "OK,
> cool, which Sunday?" I hope it will be soon like they think. I'll keep you

posted. I'll have my Dad's [Ernie's] laptop. Talk to you soon. Hey, Oh yeah, I don't want to forget. Hey Jennifer, I've been thinking about you. Are you OK? I am sure you are OK. Hi kids, I love you. Love, Cody

She emailed her Internet chatroom friend, Pete, who was also about to have surgery:

Pete, Hugs, hugs, hugs. I had to do that too this summer. I hope you're not put through the same crap I was. I think of the things I go through, or went through, and I think of you. I think of all the crap you seemed to have gone through. I am not sure, but I think so. Oh, and John is so freaked out about it all, I thought he dumped me. Nice huh? Oh well. He also felt bad and is trying to make me forgive him. I've got my health to worry about though, so hey, I'm trying to worry more about that. I hope I get to hear from you again. You're important to me, and I hope you are OK. Hey, in case you want to be in contact with me, email or call my number, and my mom will check my messages. Talk to you soon I hope. Cody

Dennis was less and less present in Cody's everyday life once she moved to her own apartment. She sometimes wondered out loud if he still cared about her. He stopped in to see her before extended overseas travel and gave her money every month. But he was rarely up to date on the details of her changing health. However, during her recent hospitalizations, Dennis had again waited in the family lounge while she was in surgery. Learning he'd done that, Cody said, "I think he really *does* care about me."

Dennis once told me he never knew what to do for fun with Cody; he thought they had so few common interests. He typically included others whenever he went out with her. But on this Wednesday evening just the two of them were together. At a restaurant on Main Street in Hopkins, they talked through the evening.

He walked her back to her apartment and told her, "It was so wonderful just talking with you tonight. I want to do this with you on a regular basis."

In her apartment, Dennis and Cody kissed goodnight, and he left. In the hallway, he paused, turned around, and went back to tell Cody how much he loved her.

THURSDAY

Cody cancelled surgery to remove her bladder stones, but not before working herself into a fever of anxiety—literally, a fever. She called me at work to report that her temperature was above 99 degrees that morning and she felt congested. The surgery nurse said operating with a fever was not advisable. Cody was off the hook. As soon as surgery was cancelled, the fever vanished and her good spirits returned.

> Hi Pete, I came down with a cold and won't be having the surgery tomorrow. I'm sorry you're probably there now. :-(. I hope everything is OK for you besides that. You can call me, and let me know you're OK. Talk to you soon. Love, Cody

FRIDAY

Each day that week, Cody made calls to Oscar, other friends, and relatives in Pennsylvania. She sent emails with loving and supportive messages. On Friday she wrote to an Internet girlfriend she'd recently had a disagreement with.

> Hey, I thought I'd email and tell you that I think about you all the time and hope you're doing OK. I don't remember much about what I said regarding us being friends. Although I know I said I didn't want to be—it's not true. If you need me any time, just let me know. I just wanted to let you know that. I'm here if you need me. Talk to you soon I hope. Love, Cody

SATURDAY

Cody awoke with a headache. She wasn't breathing comfortably, so she hooked up her BiPAP and used it for a few minutes along with oxygen. She had breakfast with John and Steve at a nearby restaurant. Ernie and I were shopping for kitchen curtains in the afternoon when Cody called Ernie's cell phone to tell us about her headache. She wasn't sure whether her eyes were sunsetting. We drove straight to her place to see for ourselves.

Cody was on the bed and the curtains were drawn. John sat on his side of the bed, looking worried. The way Cody was resting back on the pillows I could see the area on the right side of her abdomen protruding about the size of half an orange. When she sat up, it wasn't noticeable. I'd asked Cody daily if she or her PCAs saw any change from one day to the next. One attendant thought so; the other didn't. Cody thought there might be a difference, but she wasn't sure.

Her primary care doctor hadn't been too concerned about it when he examined her on Tuesday. Now that I could see it clearly, I knew the problem had to be taken care of soon, either by rescheduling bladder surgery or making an appointment with Dr. Haines to see what he thought. I fired questions at Cody and we tried to decide what to do.

"Does your headache feel like a migraine, or a shunt breakdown?"

"I don't know. I can't tell."

"Your eyes are a little wobbly, but not sunsetting. Did you take a migraine pill?"

"I couldn't find them."

I shuffled through the drawer of her bedside table and found the migraine medicine. I gave her a pill and took one for my headache, too.

Cody said, "I think I might need to go to the hospital."

I snapped at her, "I don't want to spend all night in the emergency room if this is just a migraine headache. I'll take you if you really want to go, but I won't stay."

Cody said, "That's not very supportive, Mother."

She was right, of course. I wasn't sure what to do; I was scared and frustrated with the relentless assaults on Cody's health and the decisions that had to be made. My mind raced. *Why did these things always happen on weekends? None of her doctors are reachable on weekends.* We decided to wait a little while to see if the migraine medicine worked. I told Cody to call if there was any change either way.

She asked, "Will you come back later?"

I promised, "Yes. No matter what, we'll come back to see how you're doing."

At home, Ernie and I hung kitchen curtains, and my stomach churned.

Cody had a call from Tad asking about her bladder operation. She told him she cancelled surgery. She said she had a headache, and Tad commiserated. Cody said she was so tired of health problems and didn't want more operations. Tad tried to cheer her up.

"I woke up today thinking about how adorable you were when you were born."

Cody's voice perked up. "You did?"

"Yeah, you grabbed the doctor's finger."

"I did not. I grabbed Mom's thumb."

Tad said, "Oh yeah, that's right. I remember. You grabbed her thumb so hard that she screamed 'Ouch!'"

Cody called to report that her head felt a little better. I told her we'd come by at bedtime to check on her again anyway. She told John she was pretty sure the headache was a bad migraine. She said she was so tired of headaches and worrying about operations. John put his arms around Cody and they lay still for a while.

Ernie and I came back to check on Cody around nine-thirty. Her headache was back and she had trouble looking up. Her eyes were beginning to sunset. Now we were sure. We moved into our established routine. John had already packed a change of clothing and put a handful of catheters in Cody's backpack. Ernie tucked in a few copies of the medical summary while I phoned the hospital and paged the neurosurgery resident on call.

The physician who answered was a resident who remembered Cody. I described the current situation and asked what he wanted us to do. He said he'd tell the ER we were coming, and he'd be paged when we arrived.

I said, "I have a question. In every one of these situations, Cody ends up uncomfortable, spending all night in the ER, and then has surgery sometime the next day. If that's to be the case again, would it be okay for her to stay at home to try to sleep in her own bed and come to the ER in the morning?"

The doctor said, "That would be fine. You can bring her in now, or you can wait."

I said I'd ask Cody what she wanted to do; then I asked, "Shall I call you back?"

"You don't need to. I'll be here all night. I'll tell the ER that she'll be in at some point."

Cody was scared. She knew she had to have surgery, but she said she'd rather be in her own bed than sit in an ER all night. We kissed and hugged and said a prayer for God to take care of her. I told her to call if she changed her mind or needed to go to the hospital before morning.

Sunday

The phone rang at 1:00 a.m. Cody told me she felt worse. Her voice quivered slightly when she said, "I need to go to the hospital."

"Okay, sweetie, we'll be right there."

When Ernie and I entered Cody's apartment, the lights were dim. Cody was in the same position we'd last seen her, lying back on pillows. John had just finished changing the bedding again. They both looked solemn.

Cody tried to roll onto her wheelchair but stopped. "I can't do it. I need help."

Ernie leaned down to help her transfer into her chair, but he noticed, as Cody spoke further, that she slurred her words. Our plans changed instantly. Rather than take Cody to the hospital in her van, I called 9-1-1. Ernie and I reassured Cody that it was safer to go to the hospital by ambulance. Paramedics arrived within minutes.

The November air was crisp. Cody and John spoke quietly together for a moment and hugged goodbye before she was lifted into the ambulance. I climbed in with Cody and held her hand. Her wheelchair no longer could be folded into the trunk of our car. Ernie went home for our truck to pick up her chair and meet us in the ER.

The EMT strapped down the gurney in the ambulance and tucked a blanket around Cody. He lowered the cab lights to make her more comfortable. I leaned close and kissed her cheek. As we drove to the University Hospital, the EMT made the kind of friendly conversation that sounded nothing like an emergency.

At the hospital Cody was taken to an ER cubicle and the waiting began. When Ernie arrived with her wheelchair, Cody was in terrible pain with a splitting headache. She wanted to be in her wheelchair. She kept her eyes shut as Ernie and I lifted her from the gurney to her chair. Once she was settled, Ernie told us that when he returned for the wheelchair he found John locked outside the apartment building without his key. Since it was after 1:00 a.m., he didn't want to buzz anyone to let him in. He'd waited in the cold for Ernie to return with his key.

Cody started to laugh and opened her eyes, "You mean John was stuck outside all that time?" She laughed harder and said, "Poor John!"

Ernie smiled. He and Cody exchanged I love you kisses and he went home.

The neurosurgery resident and others came in and out for the rest of the night. Tests were performed. I stayed close to Cody. I wore the lead apron and helped hold her in position for x-rays. Then we waited. The resident said he didn't want to call Dr. Haines during the night.

I stretched out on the gurney with my arm around Cody. We talked a little. With her eyes still shut, she sighed. "I thought you weren't going to stay with me."

I kissed her cheek. "Of course I'm staying with you. When have I not? We're in this together, babe. Always."

It was daylight when a nurse came to wheel Cody from the ER cubicle to a room on the fifth floor. Dr. Haines had started surgery on another patient; Cody was next. As the nurse pushed the wheelchair, Cody's arms kept falling limply to her sides. I tried to hold them up by wrapping a blanket around her. She was barely conscious.

In the fifth-floor room Cody remained in her wheelchair with her eyes closed. Her head leaned toward the side of the hospital bed. I lay on the bed with both arms around her and our faces together. She felt cold, so I tucked a second white hospital blanket around her. Cody began to talk in muffled words. She used a conversational tone, but I couldn't understand her. I strained to decipher even one word. She spoke in sentences without a sense of urgency. I asked her again and again to repeat herself. She said the same phrases several times without becoming impatient. I still didn't know what she said.

"I am so sorry that I can't understand what you're saying, but I love you."

Cody's response was slurred, but I heard her say, "I love you."

Around 9:30 a.m. a nurse came in to ask questions and fill out a form. I tucked the blanket around Cody and sat up to talk with the nurse. She directed a question to Cody and there was no response. I said, "She's been pretty out of it. We were in the ER all night."

The nurse tried to rouse Cody by pinching places on her hands and face that would normally cause someone to react. Still no response. The nurse sprang up, called a code, and the room filled with people. I stood at the foot of the bed and watched. My awareness of the next several minutes was like a series of snapshots and short video clips.

An internist entered the room and asked the group, "Who's in charge?" When no one immediately responded, she said, "Okay, then I am."

She gave instructions until the neurosurgery resident rushed in with Dr. Haines. He took over. I stood on the window side of the bed. Next to me, a resident tore open supplies he was handed. He used a 60cc syringe with a needle to extract clear fluid from the swollen area on Cody's abdomen. He filled one after another. I gathered the wrappers scattered on the sheets and threw them in the wastebasket. I wanted to help.

Dr. Haines stood over Cody's head. I saw his fingers spread across her forehead. I couldn't tell exactly what he was doing, but the gesture looked protective and gentle. He used a needle to remove cerebrospinal fluid.

The entire medical team focused on resuscitating Cody. She suddenly appeared to seize up. Her arms and legs lifted off the bed for a second. She started breathing. Dr. Haines gave follow-up instructions, and others moved closer to Cody as he walked toward the door. I followed him to the hall and asked, "Could that episode have damaged her brain? Might she be blind now from pressure on her optic nerve?"

He stopped to answer, "I don't know. We need to get a CAT scan before we do surgery." He said he'd tell me more as soon as he could. He rushed away.

A nurse I recognized from Cody's stays on the fifth floor put her hand on my arm and asked, "Is there anyone I can call for you?"

Noticing the consoling expression on her face, I thought how she must think this is a very serious situation. I was still thinking Cody was going to be fine. She was always fine—eventually. As Cody once said, she'd been on "death row" so many times.

The remaining clinicians were preparing Cody to be taken to radiology for the CAT scan, so I called Ernie. He'd been asleep; it took a minute for him to understand what I was saying.

"Cody arrested. She has to be on a respirator now. Haines is doing a CAT scan before surgery."

At first Ernie said, "Do you want me to come now or later?" Before I could answer, he said, "I'll be right there."

Cody was rolled onto the x-ray table and slid into the scanning machine. She appeared to be sleeping. I didn't need to put on a lead apron and hold her hand as I'd always done during CAT scans. She was too out of it to know I was there.

Dr. Haines called me behind the glass wall where x-ray scans of Cody's head were on monitors. The resident was with him as he described what he found. There was unexplained bleeding in Cody's brain. More than one surgery would be needed to fix the problem. The cause was not clear. I asked, "What do we do?"

Dr. Haines described some options and said Cody would go to the ICU to be prepped for surgery. I looked directly at Dr. Haines and asked, "Did I wait too long to bring her in?"

He leaned forward quickly, putting one hand on my back and the other hand on the back of his resident and said, "We'll all be second guessing this."

He must have known then; Cody's chances weren't good.

Cody was still in the ICU when Ernie arrived. Her eyes were open. She was gesturing with her right hand toward the respirator. Of course, she wanted it out.

I leaned close to her face. "You're on a respirator because you stopped breathing. You're about to go into surgery to get this fixed. Ernie and I are going home to take a shower. We'll be back by the time you're in the recovery room."

I kissed her cheek and I must have said a quick prayer. I don't remember for sure. Ernie and I went home. It didn't occur to me that I might not see her again.

I called John to tell him Cody had arrested, that she was revived now and about to have surgery. I promised to call again after she came out of recovery—business as usual. Too tired to take a shower, I fell onto the bed and into a dreamy half-sleep.

The ringing telephone pulled me awake forty-five minutes later. A woman's voice asked, "Has anyone called you?" It was the ICU nurse.

"Cody blew a pupil."

I didn't really know specifically what that meant, but I understood in my gut.

I said, "That's not good," and the nurse quickly agreed, "No, it isn't."

"Can I talk to the doctor?"

The nurse left the phone for a moment. She came back and said, "Not yet. The resident is working on her now. The doctor said he will call you back."

I told Ernie what happened and sobbed, "This is too much for her." We hugged and cried.

Doom penetrated me as I waited for Dr. Haines to call back. I couldn't sit still. I cried and paced through the house for the next twenty minutes, repeating the same prayer. *Please, God, fix her or take her. Fix her or take her. Please, God. Please don't let her suffer anymore. Please.*

When Dr. Haines called he said Cody did not revive this time. He had externalized the bottom end of the shunt through a small incision in her neck to drain spinal fluid and make sure the CSF pressure was under control. Cody was still on the respirator. Dr. Haines couldn't predict with certainly what would happen next, but he said the longer there was no change, the less likely she'd regain consciousness. He suggested we meet him in the ICU a few hours later.

I called Dennis and cried the news to him. Penelope was in England, and he was alone. We cried and talked. He said he'd come with us to see Cody and Dr. Haines. The only other call I could make was to Tad in Philadelphia. He cried with me. I promised to call again after meeting with Dr. Haines.

Ernie began tearful calls to relatives and friends who initiated phone trees of calls to others. Our grief poured. I felt weaker by the moment.

We decided not to tell John until after meeting with Dr. Haines and see-ing Cody, in case there might be some new hope by then. But tests done throughout the day showed no change.

When Dennis, Ernie, and I met with Dr. Haines, he said the situation was not good. Tests of Cody's brain function suggested she was close to brain death. He wanted to do an MRI the next morning to see how much damage to the structure of her brain there was before making any decision about life support. If the combination of tests and MRI showed severe and irreversible brain damage, we could decide to turn off the respirator.

Dennis, Ernie, and I entered the ICU room where Cody lay. There was a bandage on her head. She appeared to be asleep. She looked beautiful, but she wasn't there.

We didn't stay long; we had to talk to John.

On the way to John's apartment, Ernie called ahead and said he, Dennis, and I were stopping by for a few minutes. John said later that he had a feeling. At his apartment we sat down.

Ernie began, "It doesn't look good for Cody."

Together we told John that she had arrested again, that it looked like she was probably already brain-dead. John visibly deflated. His arms fell to his sides. His head dropped forward and he began to cry. My own breaking heart ached more.

John said he and Cody had both sensed they might not see each other again when they kissed goodbye the night before. They'd promised to love each other forever.

Monday

There was a small gathering in the conference room down the hall from the ICU on Monday. Dr. Haines and his nurse practitioner associate sat at the end of the table. Cody's partner for life and all three of her dads were present with me around the table, though Tad was there by phone from Philadelphia. Ernie held his cell phone for Tad to hear. Ernie's brother Mark waited in the family lounge while Dr. Haines spoke with us.

The MRI confirmed that Cody had severe and irreparable brain dam-age from the two respiratory arrests and brain hemorrhaging that had occurred the day before. Dr. Haines described our choices. He could do a series of brain surgeries to try to clear the extensive hemorrhaging; but, even if the operations were successful, Cody would never be able to communicate or do anything for herself again. Under these circumstances we also had the option to turn off the respirator. If Cody did not stop breathing immediately after it was removed, she'd be taken to a patient room and kept comfortable.

Without hesitation, every one of us agreed immediately; Cody would want the respirator removed. Dr. Haines insisted that we discuss it alone; he and his associate would come back in a few minutes to hear our final decision. They left the room.

I repeated the conversation and the options again to Tad on the phone. He was in complete agreement that Cody wouldn't want her body kept alive on a respirator. She'd been through enough.

Dr. Haines returned. I told him that we still unanimously and without reservation agreed with our initial decision. I was confident it was the choice Cody would make. Dr. Haines asked us to give him a moment to take out the apparatus before coming into her room.

As we walked into the ICU room, our family circled the bed where Cody lay quiet. She looked like she could have been asleep. But she was gone. She had stopped breathing the moment the respirator was removed. A monitor screen above the bed registered a continued heartbeat for the next twelve minutes as we stood around the bed crying, touching her arm or leg, or kissing her cheek. We changed places several times so that each of us could be closer to her for a few moments. John wheeled near Cody's face and held her hand. Two nurses standing in the back of the room cried, too.

Cody was gone. I was sure of it. I glanced up at the ceiling. I'd read about people with near-death experiences who floated above their bodies. But I didn't sense that Cody was there at all. I thought she had perhaps left the scene much earlier—maybe the day before. I pictured her dancing, enjoying her freedom.

That evening, Ernie and I went with John to Cody's apartment. We looked around at her unfinished projects, beadwork, bottles of medication, her clothes, piles of linens and kitchen utensils, and her extensive collection of cookware. John went up to his apartment to get ready for bed. He wanted to come back to sleep in Cody's bed, like always. Ernie and I stayed a little longer, looking at the things Cody collected, things she'd not touch again.

The telephone answering machine light was blinking. I listened to a few messages left that day. The first call was her former boyfriend Jake.

"Hi Cody, I haven't talked to you in a long time, but I thought of you today and thought I'd call to ask how you're doing."

Cody's friend Gertrude already knew what had happened, but still left a message. "Hi Cody, I know you're not there. I just wanted to hear your voice." I felt the same way.

When Ernie and I drove home late that night and pulled into the garage, Cody's empty wheelchair sat near the door. Seeing her well-worn chair without her in it was one of the hardest moments in a time filled with hard moments.

A car was parked in front of our house. Cody's last attendant, Steve, had been waiting all evening for us to come home. We invited him in.

Chapter 32

Starburst

All of Cody's parents came together to carry out the business of our daughter's death. I made the arrangements with the funeral home. Tad flew in the next day and stayed at our house. I knew Cody would want her uncle, Charlie, and cousins, Julie and Zach, to orchestrate the memorial celebration scheduled for the following Sunday.

Tad, Dennis, Penelope, Ernie, and I sorted through piles of photographs to assemble picture boards to display at the funeral home. We talked, laughed, and cried as we made our selections from photos of Cody at different stages in her life. Ernie rushed out to the copy store each time we decided on a few pictures to enlarge. We chose music from Cody's CD collection to play as people arrived for the service. James Taylor's *Never Die Young* was a given.

Dennis told me how significant the last dinner with Cody had been for him. He said he "finally got it"—that just talking with her was wonderful, easy, and enjoyable. He said he was sorry he'd not spent more time like that with her. He cried to think he "got it" only a few days before she died.

"Hey, but you got it," I said.

I wrote Cody's obituary. How to list her three dads was challenging. My first draft referred to them as "birth father, adoptive father, and stepfather." But neither Dennis nor Tad liked their labels. Tad said his made him sound more like a sperm donor. Dennis said that calling him "adoptive" father felt to him like he was letting Cody down by "qualifying" his role. "I adopted her because I loved her, and I let her down enough in life. She was my daughter. I was her father."

In the final draft, I referred to Cody's three dads as "original father, father, and stepfather." We were all fine with that.

Throughout the rest of the week, out-of-town family arrived. John's parents and both brothers came from California and stayed in his apartment. My brother Billy stayed at our house. The rest of the family stayed at nearby hotels.

Dorene told me that when she and my brother Richard drove to the funeral on Sunday, people in wheelchairs were coming from all directions on the sidewalks of downtown Hopkins. She'd thought, *I know where they're going.*

People from all parts of Cody's life came to share our goodbye to her. Art and Robbie Newberg came with all five daughters. Robbie brought snapshots of the crayon drawings on our old garage walls from when Cody starred in the *Annie* plays. Father Dan came from St. Albert's. Cody's childhood friends and neighbors, old friends and new friends joined her relatives, John's family, and the friends and colleagues of all of Cody's parents. The funeral home was so crowded that most people were standing. A few dozen guests spilled out into the hallway. I thought how much Cody would have loved to see all these people together for a big party. How unlike a party it was, without our guest of honor. Her absence was deafening.

Ernie noticed that Lewis and Orlando were stuck out in the hallway. He opened the side door and brought them in to take his spot near the front. Ernie stood next to me to the side against the wall as my brother was about to speak. I could see John crying. He sat in the front with friends in wheelchairs.

Charlie addressed the gathering with a welcome and a prayer, just as he'd done for Cody and John's Partners for Life ceremony seventeen months earlier. He prayed for a healing of our wounded hearts. Julie cried as she read scripture.

Zach said a few words, describing Cody's humor, perseverance, and warrior spirit—her way of putting others ahead of herself even in the midst of her own tough circumstances. He described her as loyal, compassionate, sensitive, joyful, and sweet. His message compared her dependence on others to our need to depend on God for eternal life. He said it was a truth that Cody knew, a faith she had. She'd said so the last time they spoke.

He reminded us, "Cody is fine. We mourn for us, the ones who miss her. If your life, your heart, your faith is in Jesus, this isn't 'Goodbye' to Cody. This is only 'See you later.'"

Charlie invited people to share stories about Cody. Dennis was the first to come forward. It amazed me that he could speak. He shared sweet and funny anecdotes. He described how he first met Cody when she was three, racing down a flight of stairs on her stomach like an alligator. He told how, at age four, she was rolled out of the recovery room after a particularly long brain surgery and said in a tremulous little voice that "it wasn't so bad." When Dennis finished he walked over to me and kissed my cheek.

Ernie was next to go to the microphone. He hadn't mentioned to me that he planned to speak. I couldn't have done it. I could not have condensed my feelings into words in the first place. I sat in tearful awe as Ernie told cute stories. He described a trick he and Cody had played on Dennis when she was in the ICU hooked up to various tubes after the final brain surgery in September to externalize her shunt. Dennis had come to stay with Cody so Ernie and I could go home to take showers. Ernie had explained about the tubing and told Dennis to make sure he didn't touch a spot he pointed to on Cody's neck. Ernie then touched the spot as though by accident and Cody feigned a realistic collapse into unconsciousness. Everyone laughed at the story. I laughed, remembering how proud I'd been that Cody played the trick so convincingly.

Tad sat still with tears streaming down his face throughout the service. Others spoke: Cody's cousins, friends, and attendant Steve. Charlie held the microphone for one of Cody's neighbors with cerebral palsy. CP affected her speech, and it was hard to catch her words. Her wailing sounds had a touching effect on us all. Several people began to cry while she spoke.

Charlie added more comforting words and Zach played the guitar and sang to Cody for the last time—"I Can Only Imagine" by Mercy Me—Cody's favorite of the songs Zach had sung to her so many times on the phone.

In all, it was a fitting celebration and precious tribute in honor of Cody's life.

After the memorial service, people who lived in Cody's building joined several PCAs and our family in the party room of Cody and John's apartment building. With help from his brother, Ernie had arranged a catered gathering. Mark, his wife Julie, and their four kids had tables of food ready by the time everyone came back from the funeral home.

Sharon wheeled toward me near the food table. Her hands twitched and her mouth strained to form the words to say how sorry she was. I thought of all the times Cody had told me what Sharon was saying when she spoke. I thanked her and said, "You and I are on our own now, Sharon. Our interpreter is gone. I'll have to work harder to be sure I know what you're saying." We laughed together for a moment. I spoke with Lewis, Orlando, Rachel, and Gertrude. Cody's cousins and her closest friends agreed to stay in touch.

The grief of friends from her building was steadfast. Another one of their own had fallen. Cody often described the shared fear and grief felt by her neighbors as they gathered in the hallway when someone in the building was taken away in an ambulance. Not knowing if their friend would return, they shared a bond and, Cody sensed, a trace of ambivalence about an attachment to someone with life-threatening medical problems. When Laura had died eighteen months before, Cody was concerned when Steve became depressed and rarely smiled. She worried that he might pull away from her when she had so many medical emergencies during the last five months. She'd recently told me, "I'm afraid he thinks I'm going to die."

After the formal gatherings were done and our relatives and friends went home, John, Ernie, and I were left to deal with Cody's possessions. John decided which of her things he wanted: the big screen TV (of course), the oak cabinetry Ernie made, wedding presents, kitchen items, and some of the artwork. I tried to select special things of Cody's to give to her friends and relatives. There was still much more.

Ernie and I loaded piles of household items, medical supplies, and craft materials into the truck to donate to an assortment of charities. The medical equipment went first. I wanted to be rid of all evidence of Cody's struggles and pain.

For the past decade Ernie had provided Cody with a new computer every two years. She researched the latest and fastest models, and he bought them for her. He replaced her keyboard when she inexplicably wore through the shift key and the letter "a." When Ernie bought her a new computer the previous year, Cody had asked him to send her old one to her Internet friend, Pete. His had crashed irreparably, and he had no money for another.

Now, I inherited Cody's newest computer and began using it for my work. I often found myself scanning through her files and directories. I felt like I was spending time with her as I looked at each message, document, or picture she cared enough to save. There were letters, a Mother's Day card she designed, sayings and prayers, medication schedules, contact lists, articles on medical conditions and latex allergies, planning lists for her commitment ceremony with John, pictures of the rings she and John gave each other, and scans of jewelry she made and gave as gifts. I found instant message exchanges with her online pal, Christopher. Their correspondence was affectionate, their conversations simple, everyday, and caring. After receiving his picture, she greeted him, "Hi Handsome." She asked about his family, worried about his health, wanted him to take care of himself, and told him he could call her anytime, day or night.

Cody's telephone now sat on the desk in my studio. Every so often I pressed the greeting button to hear her voice. She began, "Hello, this is Cody. Don't hang up!" and went on to say her number and suggest a call to her new cell phone if needed, repeating that number slowly twice before telling the caller to "have a great day." She'd lectured me often about how much she hated it when callers hung up without leaving a message. So I'd always listen until the end and leave a message, even though it made me crazy with impatience. Now, I appreciated Cody's lengthy greeting; she made me laugh.

I received wonderful sympathy cards with comments about Cody's sensitivity, insight, intelligence, humor, and especially her incredible spirit. Two weeks after Cody died I received a letter from Dr. Haines on University of Minnesota Medical School, Department of Neurosurgery letterhead:

Dear Ms. Cornell,

I wish to express my great sympathy to you and Cody's "three dads" upon her death. I have great admiration for Cody, you and all those who supported her in her remarkable life. Her spirit, her optimism, her willingness to work hard for her own healthcare, were magnificent.

We certainly wish that things could have worked out differently, but she remains an inspiring figure for all who knew her.

Sincerely,

Stephen J. Haines, MD

Lyle A. French Chair

Professor and head

On the Saturday after Thanksgiving, John, Dennis, Ernie, and I took Cody's ashes, mixed with the ashes of her dear dog Blue, to a small bridge over a body of water in South Minneapolis. The morning sky was gray. Light snowflakes floated around us as we parked the car, crossed the street and followed a paved path onto the bridge. We moved quickly and unobtrusively, so as not to draw attention to our mission. When we reached the middle of the bridge, I lifted the bag of ashes and quickly spilled them over the side. Even John could see the ashes hit the water below like a star bursting in all directions.

Epilogue

My brother Charlie said, "You sure did a great job raising Cody."

"She was a peach," I said.

Cody was a peach, a cherry, a mango, and a grape. Whenever anyone tried to credit me with her wonderfulness, I said thanks to be polite, but she was a miracle all by herself. We prayed for and experienced many miracles with Cody, never receiving the main miracle, the one where she was totally healed and could walk. But short of that, with Cody, miracles seemed to be a regular occurrence.

Charlie told me on the Christmas after she died that Cody had called on every holiday. She was the faithful connector of family and friends. I paged through my journal and read the entry I made the day Cody called to say she needed two more surgeries. By that October day, less than three weeks before she died, it had become difficult not to worry. Fear was winning. Cody and I had committed together to trust that God had a plan for us. I still couldn't believe that the plan included my losing her.

I thank God every day for letting me have Cody in my life for thirty-two years. When I'm ambushed with sorrow, I'm only sad for me. I'm truly grateful and happy for her. She's with God and has no more fear or pain. And I'm lucky. I never have to worry about my daughter again. She is forever safe.

After so many years of Cody's bubbly sweet conversation about anything and everything she happened to think of and want to share, I half expected a call from her to tell me about her arrival in heaven, how exciting it was to be met by a cheering section of her loved ones already there: my Dad, Blue, Milka, Dan, Sadie, Mort, Lorraine, Laura, and many others.

So much happens to a person in a lifetime, it's hard to know which facts or details will move a story forward and reveal the character of a life. As I relived Cody's thirty-two years, using piles of research—medical records, school records, homework, calendar notes, artwork, gifts, photographs, home movies, audiotapes, letters, her journals and my own, I was struck by how many difficult challenges she faced, one after the other. Only in recreating the timelines did I see it. That was not how Cody, or I, ever remembered the past.

I had sometimes wished for Cody's childhood back to see if I could make any part of it easier for her. Whenever I'd had those thoughts, I'd called Cody on the phone and was reminded how wonderfully well adjusted she was as an adult—still my girl, still funny, sometimes so mad or so silly, but so *her*. She assured me each time how glad she was that I did what I did, whatever it was.

Years after the fact, I learned that Cody cried at night, feeling lonely when she first moved into her own apartment at age twenty-one. I felt so sad to think of her alone and crying. But Cody had said, "I'm glad we did it exactly that way, Mom. I'm independent. A lot of my friends with disabilities never had the chance."

Cody did not see her life as one of suffering. It would be disrespectful of me to reflect back upon it that way. I admired her faith, her fighting spirit, her pure heart, and droll sense of humor in any circumstance. I don't remember the exact things we laughed about, but I mostly remember laughter, her friendship, and the magnificent feeling of being loved by her.

I thought of my daughter as color, music, fragrant flowers, and delicious fresh fruit. Cody was such a peach, and a cherry, and a mango, and a grape.

Acknowledgments

I am deeply grateful to so many who played a part in helping me transform this story into a book. I had the support of magnificent family, friends, colleagues, and publishing professionals. Most of the following fit into more than one of those groups. My sincere thanks to Cindy Brownstein and the Spina Bifida Association, Ken Atchity, Dennis Ahlburg, Beryl Singleton Bissell, Carol Carlson, Deb Carstens, Anna Charlton, Tad Cornell, Marie Demler, Bill Dorn, Dee Dunheim, Kent Eklund, Ralph Fay, Zachary Fay, Gertrude Fettig, Gary Francione, Steven Haines, Bill Hammond, Kate Havelin and colleagues in the National Writers Union, Matt Hurley, Pat Kaluza, Kathleen Kimball-Baker, John Kline, Lois and Rich Kline, Vicky Lettman, Rosanne Lombardi, Mayapriya Long, Keith Lustig, Christy Lyon, Bonnie Marsh, Kris McLain, Dorie McClelland, Julie and Geoff McWilliams, Jane Morgan, Pat Morris, Lewis and Cynthia Nixon, Paul Olson, Sharon Palay, Karen Pavlicin, Nick Pease, Anne Seltz, Shelley Shapiro, Connie Szarke, Wanda Teply, Vonnie Thomasberg, Jack Underhill, David Unowsky, Julia Washenberger, Catherine Wilson, Billie Young, and Robbie Zanko; my brothers Richard, Billy, and Charlie; to Ernie (still my hero); and most of all, thank you, Cody.

About the Author

Marly Cornell, MA, is an artist, writer, ghostwriter, and manuscript editor who worked for thirty years in the corporate nonprofit service in healthcare, behavioral services, mental health law, and physician recruitment. She coauthored, with Don Warner, *Walks on the Beach With Angie* (published in 2008 by North Star Press of St. Cloud), a finalist for a Ben Franklin Award and two Indie Excellence Awards, and the winner of two Midwest Book Awards.

Marly's only child, Cody, is the best thing that ever happened to her. As a person of faith and a social justice advocate, Marly Cornell continues to strive to be the person her dogs think she is. She lives with her husband Ernie Feil and dogs Reuben and Ricky in Minneapolis, Minnesota.

Glossary

ADD. ATTENTION DEFICIT DISORDER. A learning disability starting in childhood that causes disordered learning, inattention, and difficulty processing nervous system stimuli; can include hyperactivity and disruptive behavior.

AGORAPHOBIA. Abnormal fear, anxiety or panic brought about by feeling helpless or unable to escape a situation, resulting in an avoidance of situations associated with panicky feelings, such as large, public, or open spaces. Fear of losing control or embarrassment in public.

ALZHEIMER'S DISEASE. A brain disorder characterized by progressive memory loss and cognitive impairment; the most common form of dementia.

ANAPHYLACTIC REACTION. A severe and sometimes fatal systemic reaction (allergic response) to exposure to a specific antigen (Ex. latex, iodine, certain foods, bee sting). Previous sensitization may have included respiratory distress, swelling, itching, and hives.

ANEMIA. A deficiency of red blood cells, preventing sufficient oxygen from reaching all parts of the body.

APNEA. Cessation of breathing. (*Sleep apnea* is a disorder where breathing can slow down or stop during sleep.)

ARNOLD CHIARI MALFORMATION. A congenital anomaly wherein part of the brain protrudes down into the spinal canal, crowding the area around the brainstem; often associated with spina bifida and myelomeningocele.

AUGMENTATION CYSTOPLASTY. A reconstructive surgical procedure to increase the reservoir capacity of the bladder. Involves tissue grafts from the intestine.

BiPAP. BILATERAL POSITIVE AIRWAY PRESSURE. A BiPAP machine has plastic tubing, directing airflow into a mask to assist with breathing; often used by people with sleep apnea.

CANNULA/NASAL CANNULA. Flexible plastic tube directing oxygen into the nostrils. Tubing tucks behind ears to stay in place.

CAT SCAN/CT SCAN. Computerized axial tomography. X-ray technology that creates two-dimensional images of cross-sections of body parts. Invented in 1972.

CATHETER. A thin tube that can be inserted into the urethra to empty the bladder of urine. *See also* Foley catheter.

CEREBROSPINAL FLUID/CSF. A clear fluid that is produced by specialized cells in the brain that circulates through the ventricles of the brain and spinal cord and is reabsorbed into the blood. Its function is to maintain uniform pressure inside the brain and spinal cord.

CERVICOMEDULLARY DECOMPRESSION. Surgical procedure to remove of part of vertebrae and area of bone in the neck at the base of the skull to allow more space for the brain.

CHIROPRACTOR. Medical practitioner who uses manipulation and adjustment of musculoskeletal structures such as the spinal column to correct and improve nerve function.

COLD URTICARIA. A reactive skin disorder. Symptoms include reddening of the skin, swelling, hives and itching after skin is exposed to cold temperatures.

CONGESTIVE HEART FAILURE. A life-threatening condition in which the heart is unable to pump blood adequately for circulation throughout the body, leaving organs without sufficient oxygen and nutrients, causing organ damage.

CEREBRAL PALSY OR CP. A condition resulting from damage to the brain around the time of birth, causing disorders that affect muscle coordination, mobility, sight, speech and/or hearing.

CREDE TECHNIQUE. Using manual pressure on the bladder to express urine.

CYSTIC FIBROSIS. An inherited chronic disease in which the body produces mucus buildup that interferes with respiration and causes infections in the lungs and digestive system.

CYSTOLITHOTOMY. Surgical procedure used to remove calculus/stones from the bladder by making an incision in the bladder wall.

DALCON SHIELD. A plastic intrauterine contraceptive device (IUD) used in the early 1970s that caused user deaths, miscarriages, pelvic inflammatory disease, infection, infertility, and other complications; the subject of numerous individual lawsuits and a class action lawsuit.

DEMEROL. A prescription narcotic used to kill pain.

DIABETES. An autoimmune disorder related to the body's production and use of insulin. Increased risk of heart disease, kidney disease, nerve damage, and complications from poor circulation. Type 1, insulin-dependent diabetes, usually develops during childhood and results when the body does not produce adequate insulin. Type 2, diabetes mellitus, usually develops in adults who have an insulin deficiency or are unable to use insulin appropriately.

DIURETIC. A medication that increases urine excretion that helps reduce fluid retention.

DYSLEXIA. A learning disability in which a person has trouble interpreting written language, causing difficulty with reading, spelling and writing.

FOLEY CATHETER. A rubber catheter inserted in the urethra, with a balloon tip that is inflated to hold it in place inside the bladder. Invented in 1937.

HARRINGTON RODS. Stainless steel rods surgically placed to hold the spine in a corrected position. Used in treating scoliosis. Developed in the 1950s, first used in the 1960s.

HYDROCEPHALUS. Water on the brain. Dilation of brain ventricles due to the accumulation of cerebrospinal fluid within the skull. Increased pressure can result in an enlarged head, mental deterioration and likely, without surgical intervention, death.

HYPOVENTILATION. An inadequate ventilation of the lungs, due to shallow breathing, resulting in an abnormally high concentration of carbon dioxide in the blood and a low level of oxygen.

ILIUM. The largest pelvic bone, forming the "hip bone."

INTRACRANIAL. Inside the skull.

IUD. INTRAUTERINE DEVICE. A contraceptive device placed within the uterus to prevent conception.

IV. INTRAVENOUS. An IV needle inserted into a vein to administer medicine or nutrients.

LATEX. A plant-based protein found in rubber products and many foods. Sensitivities and allergies from latex exposure range from mild skin irritation to disability and even death.

MRI. MAGNETIC RESONANCE IMAGING. A technique using radio waves and magnetic fields to create clear images of internal body structures, especially soft tissue such as the brain and spinal cord.

MULTIPLE SCLEROSIS OR MS. An autoimmune disease affecting the central nervous system. Damaged nerve fibers in the brain result in mild to severe rates of disease progression and disability.

MYELODYSPLASIA. A group of developmental disorders of the spinal cord.

MYELOMENINGOCELE OR MENINGOMYELOCELE. A congenital defect that occurs in the first few weeks after conception. The back side of vertebrae fails to close, leaving the nerve tissue exposed; the membrane that protects the spinal cord, or the spinal cord itself, may protrude through the skin on the lower back of the spine.

MITROFANOFF. A channel created near the site of the bellybutton, often from an appendix, through which a catheter can access and drain the bladder. Often used in conjunction with a surgical bladder augmentation procedure.

NEBULIZER. A device that converts liquid medication into a fine mist that can be inhaled.

NICU. Neonatal intensive care unit.

PANIC ATTACK OR ANXIETY ATTACK. A sudden episode of intense fear lasting several minutes, accompanied by heart palpitations, dizziness, shortness of breath, and/or feelings of unreality.

PARKINSON'S DISEASE. A chronic progressive neurological disease usually in later life; linked to a decrease in the production of dopamine, causing muscle tremors, rigidity, slow movement, and problems with balance and mobility.

PCA. PERSONAL CARE ATTENDANT. An individual assisting a person with a disability in activities of daily living.

PERITONEAL FLUID. Fluid in the abdominal cavity.

PICC LINE. Peripherally inserted central catheter that allows for intravenous access for a prolonged time period.

PICU. Pediatric intensive care unit.

PNEUMONIA. Inflammation of the lungs usually caused by aspiration, virus, or infection, creating breathing difficulty and an accumulation of fluid in the lungs.

PTSD. POSTTRAUMATIC STRESS DISORDER. Recurrent symptoms including depression, anxiety, nightmares, and flashbacks that follow, often long after, a highly stressful or traumatic event.

PULMONARY HYPERTENSION. Constriction and pressure in the pulmonary arteries restricting blood flow to the lungs and causing the heart to work harder, especially on the right side; may lead to progressive heart failure.

RESTRICTIVE LUNG DISEASE. A chronic disorder that decreases the ability to expand the lung or take deep breaths, preventing intake of adequate oxygen to meet the body's needs.

SCOLIOSIS. A congenital curvature and deformity of the spine into an S or a C. Often associated with spina bifida.

SHUNT/CSF SHUNT. CEREBROSPINAL FLUID SHUNT. A flexible plastic device implanted surgically into the ventricle of the brain to divert excess cerebrospinal fluid, relieving pressure on the brain. Shunt tubing has a one-way valve directing the CSF to another area in the body to be reabsorbed into the bloodstream. *VP shunt*, ventriculoperitoneal shunt tubing leads to the abdominal cavity. *VA shunt*, ventriculoatrial shunt tubing leads into a vein near the heart.

SICKLE-CELL ANEMIA. An inherited condition wherein red blood cells change shape, clump together and sometimes block blood vessels, causing pain, organ damage, ulcerations, infection and severe anemia.

SLEEP APNEA. *See* Apnea.

SPINA BIFIDA. Open spinal column. A congenital defect in the spinal column; the spinal cord is not completely formed and may be exposed to the air in its most severe form (myelomeningocele). Occurring in the first few weeks after conception, other associated defects can include hydrocephalus, Chairi malformations, scoliosis, and problems with bowel and bladder functioning and respiration. (*See* Myelomeningocele.) Spina bifida occulta is a common and mild form of spina bifida without a protrusion from the spinal cord or its covering and often has no noticeable symptoms.

SPINAL FLUID. *See* Cerebrospinal fluid/CSF.

SUNSETTING EYES. A symptom of intracranial pressure. A limited ability or inability to raise the eyes above the midpoint or horizon, due to pressure on the optic nerve. The eyes are forced into a downcast gaze.

TUBAL LIGATION. A sterilization method involving surgery to close the fallopian tubes so that ova from the ovaries cannot pass to the uterus.

UTI. Urinary tract infection.